CKD STAGE 5

COOKBOOK

Nourishing Your Body and Supporting Kidney Health with Low Potassium, Low Sodium, and Low Phosphorus Meals with 30-Day Meal Plan

Dr Brenda White

Copyright ©Brenda White, 2024.

All rights reserved. No part of this publication may be reproduced, distributed, or transmitted in any form or by any means, including photocopying, recording, or other electronic or mechanical methods, without the prior written permission of the publisher, except for brief quotations embodied in critical reviews and specific other non-commercial uses permitted by copyright law.

Table of Contents

Introduction

Chronic kidney disease, often referred to as chronic kidney failure, is characterized by the kidneys gradually losing their ability to function properly. The main job of the kidneys is to cleanse the blood by filtering out waste and excess fluid, which is then expelled from the body in urine. When the disease reaches an advanced stage, it can lead to harmful accumulations of fluid, electrolytes, and waste in the body.

In its initial stages, chronic kidney disease may not cause any noticeable symptoms, making it possible for someone to have the disease without being aware of it until it's quite advanced.

Managing chronic kidney disease involves trying to slow down the damage to the kidneys, typically by addressing the underlying cause. However, even with proper management, the disease can continue to progress. In its most severe form, chronic kidney disease can lead to end-stage kidney failure, which can be life-threatening if not treated with dialysis or a kidney transplant.

In the United States, around 37 million people, or 15% of the population, are affected by chronic kidney disease. It often remains unnoticed and undiagnosed until it has significantly progressed.

Certain ethnic groups, including African Americans, Hispanics, Native Americans, and Asian Americans, are at a higher risk of developing chronic kidney disease compared to white individuals, possibly due to healthcare disparities.

As kidney disease progresses, waste can accumulate quickly in the body. The goal of treatment is to halt or slow down the worsening of kidney function by managing the root cause.

Stage 1: A person with stage 1 chronic kidney disease has a GFR (glomerular filtration rate) of 90 ml/min per 1.73 m2 or higher, indicating normal kidney function but with signs of kidney damage, such as protein in the urine or physical damage to the kidneys.

Stage 2: The GFR is between 60 and 89 ml/min per 1.73 m2. While this suggests the kidneys are still functioning well, there are additional indications of kidney damage.

Stage 3: This stage is split into two sub-stages:

- **Stage 3a:** With a GFR of 45–59 ml/min per 1.73 m2.
- **Stage 3b:** With a GFR of 30–44 ml/min per 1.73 m2.

Symptoms might include swelling in hands and feet, back pain, more frequent urination, anemia, high blood pressure, and bone disease.

People with stages 1 to 3 can potentially slow kidney damage by controlling blood sugar and blood pressure, eating healthily, avoiding tobacco, staying active, keeping a moderate weight, and consulting with a kidney specialist.

Stage 4: Here, the GFR drops to 15–29 ml/min per 1.73 m2, indicating moderate to severe kidney damage. It's a critical stage that precedes kidney failure, and symptoms and complications become more common.

Stage 5: This final stage is characterized by a GFR of less than 15 ml/min per 1.73 m2, meaning the kidneys are failing or close to it. Symptoms of kidney failure include itching, muscle cramps, nausea, vomiting, swelling, back pain, frequent urination, sleep difficulties, and trouble breathing. Treatment at this stage requires dialysis or a kidney transplant to help filter the blood since the kidneys can no longer do so effectively.

Signs and Symptoms

As chronic kidney disease progresses gradually, the signs and symptoms may take time to appear. The slow deterioration of kidney function can lead to the accumulation of fluids, waste, and electrolyte imbalances. The severity of kidney function loss can lead to various issues, such as:

- Feeling nauseous
- Throwing up
- A decrease in hunger
- Tiredness and a lack of energy

- Trouble sleeping
- Changes in how often you pee
- Less mental clarity
- High blood pressure that resists treatment
- Breathlessness if fluid accumulates in the lungs
- Chest discomfort if fluid surrounds the heart
- Puffiness around the eyes
- Swollen legs
- Persistent breathlessness
- Unintentional weight reduction
- Breath that smells like urine
- Tingling in your hands and feet
- Easy bruising or bleeding
- Pain in the bones
- Alterations in skin, hair, or nails
- Feeling sleepy or mentally foggy
- Problems with sexual function
- Persistent itching
- Muscle spasms and cramps
- Blood in your stool
- Persistent hiccups
- Excessive thirst
- Reduced sexual interest

Causes

Several diseases and conditions can lead to chronic kidney disease, including:

- Diabetes (both type 1 and type 2)
- Persistent high blood pressure
- Glomerulonephritis, which is swelling of the kidney's filters
- Interstitial nephritis, which is inflammation of the kidney's tubules and surrounding areas
- Hereditary kidney conditions like polycystic kidney disease
- Long-term blockage of the urinary tract from conditions like enlarged prostate, kidney stones, or some cancers
- Vesicoureteral reflux, a condition causing urine to back up into your kidneys

- Repeated kidney infections

Risk Factors

Several factors can raise your chances of developing chronic kidney disease:

- Diabetes
- High blood pressure
- Cardiovascular disease
- Smoking
- Excess weight
- Ethnic backgrounds such as Black, Native American, or Asian American
- A family history of kidney issues
- Abnormal kidney structure
- Advancing age
- Regular use of medications that may harm the kidneys
- Cigarette use
- High cholesterol levels
- Autoimmune diseases
- Obstructive kidney disease, including complications from benign prostatic hyperplasia
- Atherosclerosis
- Liver conditions like cirrhosis
- Narrowing of the kidney-supplying artery
- Kidney or bladder cancer
- Kidney stones or infections
- Conditions like systemic lupus erythematosus
- Diseases like scleroderma or vasculitis
- Vesicoureteral reflux, where urine flows backward into the kidney

Complications

Kidney disease can have a wide-ranging impact on your body. Here are some issues it might cause:

- Swelling in your limbs and high blood pressure due to fluid buildup, or even fluid in your lungs
- Dangerous spikes in your blood's potassium levels, which can harm your heart and be serious.
- Anemia, which means your blood doesn't have enough red cells
- Heart problems

- Weaker bones and a higher chance of breaking them
- A drop in your sex drive, trouble with getting an erection, or fertility issues
- Brain and nerve issues that can lead to trouble focusing, personality shifts, or seizures
- A weaker immune system, making you more prone to catching bugs
- Inflammation around your heart called pericarditis
- Risks during pregnancy for both mom and baby
- Kidney failure that's so bad you might need dialysis or a new kidney to stay alive

Prevention

- **Be smart with over-the-counter meds:** Stick to the recommended doses for things like aspirin, ibuprofen, and acetaminophen to avoid hurting your kidneys.
- **Keep your weight in a healthy range:** Stay active to maintain or get to a weight that's good for you.
- **Quit smoking:** It's bad news for your kidneys, and if you need a hand stopping, there's help there from support groups to meds.
- Team up with your doctor to manage any conditions that could hurt your kidneys.

Ten ways to manage kidney disease

- Keep your blood pressure in check
- If you've got diabetes, manage your blood sugar
- Regularly check your kidney health with your healthcare team
- Take your meds as they're prescribed
- Plan your meals with a dietitian's help
- Make exercise a regular thing
- Aim for a healthy weight
- Get plenty of sleep
- Stop smoking
- Find good ways to deal with stress and feeling down

What If My Kidneys Fail?

While some individuals manage to live with kidney disease for many years and keep their kidney function stable, others may experience a rapid decline leading to kidney failure.

Kidney failure occurs when the kidneys can no longer perform their duties effectively, operating at less than 15 percent of their normal capacity. At this stage, waste products and excess fluid may accumulate in the body, potentially causing various symptoms.

To replace your lost kidney function, you may have one of three treatment options:

- Hemodialysis
- Peritoneal dialysis
- Kidney transplant
- Managing end-stage renal disease (ESRD) with dialysis or a transplant

Some kids with kidney failure might opt out of dialysis or transplantation and instead focus on managing their condition with the support of their healthcare team, medications, and careful attention to diet and lifestyle.

Treatment Options

The treatment for chronic kidney disease (CKD) depends on its severity.

The primary approaches include:

- Lifestyle modifications to keep as healthy as possible
- Medications to address problems like high blood pressure and cholesterol
- Dialysis to mimic kidney function, often needed in stage 5 CKD
- Kidney transplant, which might be necessary for stage 5 CKD

Kidney Disease in Children

How often does kidney disease occur in kids?

Kidney disease isn't very common in children, and it's hard to pinpoint the exact number affected since many don't show symptoms in the early stages.

Which kids are more likely to get kidney disease?

Boys are more likely to have CKD than girls. In North America, Black children face a two to three times higher risk of developing CKD compared to white children.

What complications can arise from kidney disease in kids?

Some of the complications include:

- Anemia
- Heart disease
- Imbalances in blood electrolytes, like potassium
- Growth issues, such as being shorter than average
- High blood pressure
- Infections
- Metabolic acidosis
- Mineral and bone disorders
- Cognitive difficulties
- Urinary incontinence

What are the signs of kidney disease in kids?

Early-stage kidney disease might not cause any symptoms in children. But as it progresses, the signs can include:

- Swelling in the feet, legs, hands, or face (edema)
- Changes in urine output, possibly needing to pee more often or bedwetting
- Foamy urine from excess protein (proteinuria)
- Pink or cola-colored urine due to blood presence (hematuria)

Other possible symptoms are:

- Decreased appetite
- Fatigue
- Fevers
- High blood pressure
- Itchy skin
- Nausea or vomiting
- Shortness of breath
- Difficulty concentrating
- Weakness
- Weight loss
- Stunted growth

These symptoms can vary based on the underlying cause of the kidney disease.

Kidney disease in children can result from:

- Birth defects
- Genetic conditions
- Infections
- Nephrotic syndrome
- Systemic diseases
- Trauma
- Urinary blockages or reflux

Living with Stage 5 CKD

In stage 5 of chronic kidney disease (CKD), the kidneys can't manage fluid levels properly, leading to a buildup of toxins and water in the body. A blood test at this stage shows an estimated glomerular filtration rate (eGFR) below 15 ml/min, indicating severely reduced kidney function. This stage often comes with other health issues like anemia and bone problems due to the kidneys' inability to perform their normal functions.

At this point, it's necessary to start kidney replacement therapy, which includes dialysis or a kidney transplant, or to consider conservative care. The kidneys have sustained permanent damage and can't filter waste or excess water effectively anymore, so another method to remove these is required.

For someone with stage 5 CKD, also known as end-stage renal disease (ESRD), the kidneys have nearly lost all their filtering ability, and survival depends on dialysis or a kidney transplant.

Symptoms of Stage 5 CKD

Symptoms of stage 5 CKD can include a loss of appetite, nausea, headaches, fatigue, difficulty concentrating, itching, producing little to no urine, swelling (especially around the eyes and ankles), muscle cramps, tingling in the hands or feet, skin color changes, and increased skin pigmentation. These symptoms arise because the kidneys can't remove waste and fluids from the body, leading to a buildup of toxins in the blood.

Dialysis treatments for people with stage 5 CKD

People often feel much better after starting dialysis, as it helps remove the toxins from the blood and replaces some functions the kidneys can't perform anymore, allowing for a better quality of life. There are two types of dialysis:

1. **Hemodialysis,** which can be done at a center or home with a helper. It uses a machine to filter a small amount of blood through a dialyzer, or artificial kidney, to remove toxins.
2. **Peritoneal dialysis (PD)**, which is needle-free and can be done at home or work without a helper.

Kidney transplant option

If you're interested in a kidney transplant, let your kidney doctor know. They'll explain how to get on a waiting list for a deceased donor kidney or find a living donor.

When at stage 5 CKD, either dialysis or a kidney transplant is necessary to continue living.

A healthy diet for stage 5 CKD

- Enjoying a variety of grains, fruits, and veggies, but being mindful to limit or skip those high in phosphorus or potassium.
- Choosing foods low in saturated fats and cholesterol, and keeping total fats moderate, particularly if you're managing high cholesterol, diabetes, or heart issues.
- Cutting back on overly processed foods rich in sodium and opting for less salt in cooking.
- Striving for a healthy weight by eating enough calories and staying active as much as you're able.
- Reducing calcium intake if needed.
- Watching how much you drink.
- Upping your protein intake as recommended by your dietitian to make up for what's lost during dialysis.
- Taking special kidney-friendly vitamins that are rich in water-soluble B vitamins and have no more than 100 mg of vitamin C.
- Personalize your intake of vitamin D and iron based on your specific needs.

Steps to take at stage 5 kidney disease

1. Regular check-ins with your kidney specialist to monitor your health and track the disease's progression. Keep up with appointments with your primary care physician and other specialists to stay on top of any other health issues.
2. Sticking to a kidney-friendly diet, might mean watching how much potassium, phosphorus, sodium, or fluids you have. If you're about to start dialysis, your diet may need some tweaks. Chat with your renal dietitian about the best food choices for you so you can feel your best.
3. Discuss your health insurance with your insurance coordinator to ensure you've got the best coverage. Before tweaking your plan, get their advice to understand your options.
4. Getting ready for treatment, whether that's setting up your space for home dialysis or getting familiar with your local dialysis center if you're going in-center.
5. Building a support network of friends, family, and your healthcare team who can offer you the support you need.

Questions to ask your doctor about stage 5 kidney disease

What should I expect from treatment for kidney failure?

Explore the various treatments with your doctor to find what suits your lifestyle, whether it's a transplant, home dialysis, or in-center dialysis.

Am I eligible for a kidney transplant, and what steps should I take?

Discuss your eligibility for a transplant with your nephrologist and start planning and searching for a donor early.

How can I manage dialysis around my work schedule?

Work with your nephrologist to figure out a dialysis schedule that fits your lifestyle and health needs. Home dialysis options might offer more flexibility.

Do I need to adjust any medications I'm currently taking?

Review all your medications, including vitamins and supplements, with your doctor to ensure they're safe to continue with your treatment.

Stage 5 kidney failure life expectancy

Having end-stage renal disease (ESRD) doesn't mean it's the end of your life. Your life expectancy with ESRD can vary based on your treatment choices and overall health. Remember, with today's treatments, you can live a fulfilling life for many years. There's no cure for kidney disease and the damage can't be reversed, but treatments are available to help you live well for a long time.

Complications of advanced kidney disease

- Swelling due to fluid buildup in various body parts.
- Anemia, which means a lower level of red blood cells.
- Hyperkalemia, a condition where high potassium levels can harm your heart.
- Cardiovascular issues affecting your heart and blood vessels.
- Decreased libido.
- Challenges with erectile function.
- Weakened bones, known as osteomalacia.
- Potential harm to your central nervous system.
- A compromised immune system.

Building a CKD-Friendly Pantry

Foods Containing More Sodium:

- Processed meats such as bacon, corned beef, ham, hot dogs, luncheon meats, and sausages
- Condensed and instant soups, bouillon cubes, and ramen noodle packs
- Pre-packaged mixes for dishes like hamburgers and pancakes
- Preserved vegetables, vegetable juices, and canned beans, chicken, fish, and meats
- Tomato-based products such as canned tomatoes and tomato juice
- Cottage cheese
- Frozen prepared meals
- Vegetables with added sauces in frozen form
- Pickled items including olives, pickles, and relishes
- Snack foods like pretzels, chips, crackers, and salted nuts
- Boxed meals and side dishes that are ready to eat
- Dressings for salads, bottled condiments, and marinades
- Salt and flavored salts like garlic salt
- Pre-mixed seasonings and sauce packets
- Certain ready-to-eat cereals, baked goods, and bread
- Soy sauce

Foods Containing Less Sodium:

- Popcorn made by air-popping
- Cooked cereals without any added salt
- Fresh cuts of meat, poultry, and seafood
- Fresh or frozen produce
- Frozen dinners, peanut butter, and salad dressings with reduced sodium
- Cheeses that are low in fat and sodium
- Rice and noodles without added salt
- Nuts that are not salted

Foods With Higher Potassium Content:

- Various fruits such as fresh apricots, bananas, cantaloupe, dates, kiwi, nectarines, oranges and their juice, prunes and prune juice, raisins
- An array of vegetables including acorn and butternut squash, avocados, baked beans, various greens like beets, cooked broccoli, cooked brussels sprouts, chard, chili peppers, cooked mushrooms, potatoes, pumpkin, cooked spinach, legumes such as split peas, lentils, and beans, sweet potatoes and yams, tomatoes in various forms such as juice and sauce, and vegetable juice

Foods With Lower Potassium Content:

- Fruits like apples and their juice, canned apricots and apricot nectar, various berries, cranberry juice, fruit cocktails, grapefruit, grapes and grape juice, lemons, limes, papayas, peaches, pears, pineapple, plums, rhubarb, tangerines, watermelon
- Vegetables such as alfalfa sprouts, canned bamboo shoots, bell peppers, fresh broccoli, cabbage, carrots, cauliflower, raw celery and onions, corn, cucumber, eggplant, green beans, kale, lettuce, fresh mushrooms, okra, cooked summer squash

Foods Rich in Phosphorus:

- Legumes like beans, lentils, nuts
- Bran cereals and oatmeal
- Certain beverages such as cola and some bottled iced teas
- Dairy products including milk, cheese, and yogurt
- Ice cream
- Processed meats like hot dogs and canned meats

Foods Low in Phosphorus:

- Corn and rice-based cereals
- A variety of fresh fruits and vegetables
- Home-brewed iced tea
- Rice milk that is not enriched
- Sorbet
- Meats that are not processed

Protein Substitutions

High-Phosphorus or High-Potassium Proteins

- **Substitute Red Meat** (beef, pork) with:

    - **Skinless Chicken Breast**: Lower in phosphorus and potassium.

    - **Fish** (like cod or tilapia): Lower in phosphorus and provides healthy omega-3 fatty acids.

    - **Tofu**: A versatile, plant-based protein that's kidney-friendly when prepared properly.

Dairy Products

- **Substitute Whole Milk** with:

    - **Unsweetened Almond Milk**: Lower in potassium and phosphorus.

    - **Rice Milk**: Another low-potassium and low-phosphorus option.

Cheese

- **Substitute High-Phosphorus Cheeses** (like cheddar) with:

    - **Low-sodium ricotta or Cottage Cheese**: Use in moderation and choose lower-sodium varieties.

Grain and Starch Substitutions

High-Phosphorus Whole Grains

- **Substitute Brown Rice and Whole Wheat Bread** with:

    - **White Rice**: Lower in potassium and phosphorus.

    - **White Bread**: Lower in phosphorus; look for low-sodium options.

    - **Rice Cakes**: A good low-phosphorus and low-potassium snack option.

High-Potassium Cereals

- **Substitute Bran Cereals** with:

    - **Cornflakes or Rice Krispies**: Lower in potassium and phosphorus.

Vegetable Substitutions

High-Potassium Vegetables

- **Substitute Potatoes and Sweet Potatoes** with:
    - **Cauliflower**: Can be used to make a mash or rice substitute.
    - **Zucchini**: Great for roasting, grilling, or adding to salads.
- **Substitute Spinach and Swiss Chard** with:
    - **Kale**: Lower in potassium when cooked.
    - **Lettuce**: Such as romaine or iceberg, for salads and sandwiches.

Tomato Products

- **Substitute Tomato Sauce** with:
    - **Red Bell Pepper Puree**: Provides a similar texture and sweetness without the high potassium.
    - **Low-Potassium Marinara Sauce**: Make your own using peeled, deseeded tomatoes and red bell peppers.

Fruit Substitutions

High-Potassium Fruits

- **Substitute Bananas and Oranges** with:
    - **Apples**: Fresh, peeled, or as applesauce.
    - **Berries**: Blueberries, strawberries, and raspberries are great low-potassium options.

Beverage Substitutions

High-Potassium Juices

- **Substitute Orange Juice and Prune Juice** with:
    - **Apple Juice**: Lower in potassium and phosphorus.
    - **Cranberry Juice**: Good for kidney health when consumed in moderation.

High-Sodium Broths

- **Substitute Regular Chicken or Beef Broth** with:

    - **Low-Sodium Broth**: Homemade or store-bought varieties with reduced sodium content.

    - **Vegetable Broth**: Make your own with low-potassium vegetables.

Snack Substitutions

Salty Snacks

- **Substitute Potato Chips and Pretzels** with:

    - **Unsalted Popcorn**: A great low-sodium snack.

    - **Fresh Vegetables**: Carrot sticks, cucumber slices, and bell pepper strips with a CKD-friendly dip.

Sweet Treats

- **Substitute High-Sugar Desserts** with:

    - **Fresh Fruit Salad**: Use low-potassium fruits.

    - **Chia Seed Pudding**: Made with unsweetened almond milk and fresh berries.

Cooking and Seasoning Substitutions

High-Sodium Seasonings

- **Substitute Table Salt and Soy Sauce** with:

    - **Herbs and Spices**: Garlic powder, onion powder, basil, parsley, thyme, and rosemary.

    - **Salt-Free Seasoning Blends**: Such as Mrs. Dash or homemade blends.

    - **Lemon Juice or Vinegar**: For adding acidity and enhancing flavors without sodium.

High-Sodium Sauces

- **Substitute Store-Bought Salad Dressings and Marinades** with:

    - **Homemade Vinaigrettes**: Using olive oil, vinegar, and herbs.

- **Greek Yogurt-Based Dressings**: Lower in sodium and can be flavored with herbs and spices.

Tips for making healthy food choices

- Spice things up instead of using salt.
- Pile veggies like spinach, broccoli, and peppers on your pizza.
- Bake or broil your meat and fish instead of frying.
- Skip the gravy and extra fats.
- Cut back on added sugars.
- Work your way from whole milk to skim or low-fat.
- Go for whole grains like whole wheat bread, brown rice, and oats.
- Read labels to pick foods low in bad fats, salt, and sugar.
- Snack slowly—try popcorn over cake, or an orange over juice.
- Track what you eat for a week to spot when you might overdo it with high-fat or high-calorie foods.

Meal Planning

Day 1

Breakfast: Poached Eggs on Avocado Toast
Lunch: Lentil and Vegetable Soup with Whole Grain Crackers
Dinner: Grilled Chicken Kebabs with Bell Peppers and Zucchini

Day 2

Breakfast: Overnight Oats with Peanut Butter and Raspberries
Lunch: Tuna Salad Stuffed Tomatoes
Dinner: Baked Salmon with Roasted Sweet Potatoes and Green Beans

Day 3

Breakfast: Baked Oats with Blueberries
Lunch: Quinoa and Roasted Vegetable Bowl with Tahini Dressing
Dinner: Lentil and Vegetable Curry over Cauliflower Rice

Day 4

Breakfast: Egg White Frittata with Spinach and Feta
Lunch: Grilled Salmon and Asparagus Foil Packets
Dinner: Grilled Pork Tenderloin with Roasted Apples and Onions

Day 5

Breakfast: Quinoa Porridge with Stewed Apples and Cinnamon
Lunch: Chickpea and Cucumber Salad with Lemon Vinaigrette
Dinner: Quinoa and Black Bean Stuffed Bell Peppers

Day 6

Breakfast: Avocado and Tomato Toast with Chia Seeds
Lunch: Turkey and Avocado Lettuce Wraps
Dinner: Baked Tilapia with Roasted Broccoli and Garlic

Day 7

Breakfast: Scrambled Tofu with Bell Peppers and Mushrooms
Lunch: Roasted Butternut Squash and Kale Salad with Pumpkin Seeds
Dinner: Tofu and Vegetable Stir-Fry with Brown Rice Noodles

Day 8

Breakfast: Chia Pudding with Mango and Coconut Milk
Lunch: Lentil and Sweet Potato Shepherd's Pie
Dinner: Grilled Shrimp Skewers with Mango Salsa and Cauliflower Rice

Day 9

Breakfast: Zucchini Fritters with Poached Eggs
Lunch: Lentil and Kale Soup with Whole Grain Bread
Dinner: Baked Chicken Parmesan with Zucchini Noodles

Day 10

Breakfast: Oatmeal Pancakes with Blueberry Compote
Lunch: Chicken and Vegetable Soup with Whole Grain Crackers
Dinner: Lentil and Sweet Potato Curry with Cauliflower Rice

Day 11

Breakfast: Poached Eggs on Avocado Toast
Lunch: Lentil and Vegetable Soup with Whole Grain Crackers
Dinner: Grilled Chicken Kebabs with Bell Peppers and Zucchini

Day 12

Breakfast: Overnight Oats with Peanut Butter and Raspberries
Lunch: Tuna Salad Stuffed Tomatoes
Dinner: Baked Salmon with Roasted Sweet Potatoes and Green Beans

Day 13

Breakfast: Baked Oats with Blueberries
Lunch: Quinoa and Roasted Vegetable Bowl with Tahini Dressing
Dinner: Lentil and Vegetable Curry over Cauliflower Rice

Day 14

Breakfast: Egg White Frittata with Spinach and Feta
Lunch: Grilled Salmon and Asparagus Foil Packets
Dinner: Grilled Pork Tenderloin with Roasted Apples and Onions

Day 15

Breakfast: Quinoa Porridge with Stewed Apples and Cinnamon
Lunch: Chickpea and Cucumber Salad with Lemon Vinaigrette
Dinner: Quinoa and Black Bean Stuffed Bell Peppers

Day 16

Breakfast: Avocado and Tomato Toast with Chia Seeds
Lunch: Turkey and Avocado Lettuce Wraps
Dinner: Baked Tilapia with Roasted Broccoli and Garlic

Day 17

Breakfast: Scrambled Tofu with Bell Peppers and Mushrooms
Lunch: Roasted Butternut Squash and Kale Salad with Pumpkin Seeds
Dinner: Tofu and Vegetable Stir-Fry with Brown Rice Noodles

Day 18

Breakfast: Chia Pudding with Mango and Coconut Milk
Lunch: Lentil and Sweet Potato Shepherd's Pie
Dinner: Grilled Shrimp Skewers with Mango Salsa and Cauliflower Rice

Day 19

Breakfast: Zucchini Fritters with Poached Eggs
Lunch: Lentil and Kale Soup with Whole Grain Bread
Dinner: Baked Chicken Parmesan with Zucchini Noodles

Day 20

Breakfast: Oatmeal Pancakes with Blueberry Compote
Lunch: Chicken and Vegetable Soup with Whole Grain Crackers
Dinner: Lentil and Sweet Potato Curry with Cauliflower Rice

Day 21

Breakfast: Poached Eggs on Avocado Toast
Lunch: Lentil and Vegetable Soup with Whole Grain Crackers
Dinner: Grilled Chicken Kebabs with Bell Peppers and Zucchini

Day 22

Breakfast: Overnight Oats with Peanut Butter and Raspberries
Lunch: Tuna Salad Stuffed Tomatoes
Dinner: Baked Salmon with Roasted Sweet Potatoes and Green Beans

Day 23

Breakfast: Baked Oats with Blueberries
Lunch: Quinoa and Roasted Vegetable Bowl with Tahini Dressing
Dinner: Lentil and Vegetable Curry over Cauliflower Rice

Day 24

Breakfast: Egg White Frittata with Spinach and Feta
Lunch: Grilled Salmon and Asparagus Foil Packets
Dinner: Grilled Pork Tenderloin with Roasted Apples and Onions

Day 25

Breakfast: Quinoa Porridge with Stewed Apples and Cinnamon
Lunch: Chickpea and Cucumber Salad with Lemon Vinaigrette
Dinner: Quinoa and Black Bean Stuffed Bell Peppers

Day 26

Breakfast: Avocado and Tomato Toast with Chia Seeds
Lunch: Turkey and Avocado Lettuce Wraps
Dinner: Baked Tilapia with Roasted Broccoli and Garlic

Day 27

Breakfast: Scrambled Tofu with Bell Peppers and Mushrooms
Lunch: Roasted Butternut Squash and Kale Salad with Pumpkin Seeds
Dinner: Tofu and Vegetable Stir-Fry with Brown Rice Noodles

Day 28

Breakfast: Chia Pudding with Mango and Coconut Milk
Lunch: Lentil and Sweet Potato Shepherd's Pie
Dinner: Grilled Shrimp Skewers with Mango Salsa and Cauliflower Rice

Day 29

Breakfast: Zucchini Fritters with Poached Eggs
Lunch: Lentil and Kale Soup with Whole Grain Bread
Dinner: Baked Chicken Parmesan with Zucchini Noodles

Day 30

Breakfast: Oatmeal Pancakes with Blueberry Compote
Lunch: Chicken and Vegetable Soup with Whole Grain Crackers
Dinner: Lentil and Sweet Potato Curry with Cauliflower Rice

Breakfast

Poached Eggs on Avocado Toast

Prep Time: 10 minutes | **Cook Time:** 5 minutes | **Total Time:** 15 minutes | **Per Serving:** 2 servings

Ingredients:

- 2 large eggs

- 2 slices whole grain bread

- 1 ripe avocado

- 1/2 lemon, juiced

- Salt and pepper, to taste

- Red pepper flakes (optional)

Instructions:

1. Bring a pot of water to a gentle simmer. Add a splash of vinegar if desired.

2. Crack each egg into a small bowl, then gently slide into the simmering water.

3. Cook eggs for about 3-4 minutes, or until whites are set but yolks are runny.

4. While eggs are cooking, toast the bread slices.

5. In a bowl, mash the avocado with lemon juice, salt, and pepper.

6. Spread the mashed avocado evenly on each slice of toast.

7. Using a slotted spoon, carefully remove the poached eggs from the water and place them on top of the avocado toast.

8. Sprinkle with red pepper flakes if desired and serve immediately.

Nutritional Value: Calories: 250 | Protein: 12g | Carbohydrates: 22g | Fats: 15g | Sodium: 150mg | Potassium: 450mg | Fiber: 6g

Overnight Oats with Peanut Butter and Raspberries

Prep Time: 5 minutes | **Cook Time:** 0 minutes | **Total Time:** 5 minutes + overnight | **Per Serving:** 2 servings

Ingredients:

- 1 cup rolled oats

- 1 cup unsweetened almond milk

- 2 tablespoons peanut butter

- 1/2 cup fresh raspberries

- 1 tablespoon chia seeds

- 1 teaspoon honey (optional)

Instructions:

1. In a bowl or jar, combine rolled oats, almond milk, peanut butter, chia seeds, and honey if using.

2. Stir well to combine.

3. Cover and refrigerate overnight.

4. In the morning, give the oats a good stir.

5. Top with fresh raspberries before serving.

Nutritional Value: Calories: 300 | Protein: 10g | Carbohydrates: 40g | Fats: 12g | Sodium: 150mg | Potassium: 350mg | Fiber: 8g

Baked Oats with Blueberries

Prep Time: 10 minutes | **Cook Time:** 30 minutes | **Total Time:** 40 minutes | **Per Serving:** 4 servings

Ingredients:

- 2 cups rolled oats

- 1 cup unsweetened almond milk

- 1/2 cup fresh blueberries

- 1/4 cup maple syrup

- 1 teaspoon vanilla extract

- 1 teaspoon baking powder

- 1/2 teaspoon cinnamon

- Pinch of salt

Instructions:

1. Preheat oven to 350°F (175°C).

2. In a large bowl, mix the oats, almond milk, maple syrup, vanilla extract, baking powder, cinnamon, and salt.

3. Fold in the blueberries.

4. Pour the mixture into a greased baking dish.

5. Bake for 30 minutes or until the top is golden brown and the oats are set.

6. Allow to cool slightly before serving.

Nutritional Value: Calories: 250 | Protein: 6g | Carbohydrates: 45g | Fats: 5g | Sodium: 200mg | Potassium: 150mg | Fiber: 5g

Egg White Frittata with Spinach and Feta

Prep Time: 10 minutes | **Cook Time:** 20 minutes | **Total Time:** 30 minutes | **Per Serving:** 4 servings

Ingredients:

- 8 egg whites

- 1 cup fresh spinach, chopped

- 1/4 cup feta cheese, crumbled

- 1/4 cup diced onion

- 1 tablespoon olive oil

- Salt and pepper, to taste

Instructions:

1. Preheat oven to 375°F (190°C).

2. In an oven-safe skillet, heat olive oil over medium heat.

3. Add diced onion and sauté until translucent.

4. Add chopped spinach and cook until wilted.

5. In a bowl, whisk the egg whites with salt and pepper.

6. Pour the egg whites over the spinach and onion mixture.

7. Sprinkle feta cheese on top.

8. Cook on the stovetop until the edges begin to set, then transfer the skillet to the oven.

9. Bake for 10-15 minutes, or until the frittata is fully set.

10. Slice and serve warm.

Nutritional Value: Calories: 120 | Protein: 14g | Carbohydrates: 3g | Fats: 6g | Sodium: 200mg | Potassium: 250mg | Fiber: 1g

Quinoa Porridge with Stewed Apples and Cinnamon

Prep Time: 10 minutes | **Cook Time:** 20 minutes | **Total Time:** 30 minutes | **Per Serving:** 2 servings

Ingredients:

- 1 cup cooked quinoa

- 1 cup unsweetened almond milk

- 1 apple, peeled and diced

- 1 tablespoon maple syrup

- 1 teaspoon cinnamon

- 1/2 teaspoon vanilla extract

- Pinch of salt

Instructions:

1. In a saucepan, combine diced apple, maple syrup, and cinnamon. Cook over medium heat until apples are tender, about 10 minutes.

2. In another saucepan, combine cooked quinoa, almond milk, vanilla extract, and salt. Heat over medium heat until warm, stirring occasionally.

3. Divide quinoa porridge into bowls and top with stewed apples.

4. Serve warm.

Nutritional Value: Calories: 220 | Protein: 6g | Carbohydrates: 42g | Fats: 4g | Sodium: 100mg | Potassium: 200mg | Fiber: 5g

Avocado and Tomato Toast with Chia Seeds

Prep Time: 5 minutes | **Cook Time:** 0 minutes | **Total Time:** 5 minutes | **Per Serving:** 2 servings

Ingredients:

- 2 slices whole grain bread

- 1 ripe avocado

- 1/2 cup cherry tomatoes, halved

- 1 tablespoon chia seeds

- 1/2 lemon, juiced

- Salt and pepper, to taste

Instructions:

1. Toast the whole grain bread slices.

2. In a bowl, mash the avocado with lemon juice, salt, and pepper.

3. Spread the mashed avocado evenly on the toast.

4. Top with cherry tomatoes and sprinkle with chia seeds.

5. Serve immediately.

Nutritional Value: Calories: 220 | Protein: 5g | Carbohydrates: 26g | Fats: 12g | Sodium: 150mg | Potassium: 400mg | Fiber: 8g

Scrambled Tofu with Bell Peppers and Mushrooms

Prep Time: 10 minutes | **Cook Time:** 10 minutes | **Total Time:** 20 minutes | **Per Serving:** 2 servings

Ingredients:

- 1 block of firm tofu, drained and crumbled
- 1/2 bell pepper, diced
- 1/2 cup mushrooms, sliced
- 1/4 cup diced onion
- 1 tablespoon olive oil
- 1 teaspoon turmeric
- Salt and pepper, to taste

Instructions:

1. In a skillet, heat olive oil over medium heat.
2. Add diced onion and bell pepper, and sauté until softened.
3. Add sliced mushrooms and cook until tender.
4. Add crumbled tofu to the skillet, along with turmeric, salt, and pepper.
5. Cook, stirring frequently, until tofu is heated through and evenly coated with spices.
6. Serve warm.

Nutritional Value: Calories: 180 | Protein: 14g | Carbohydrates: 8g | Fats: 10g | Sodium: 180mg | Potassium: 300mg | Fiber: 4g

Chia Pudding with Mango and Coconut Milk

Prep Time: 10 minutes | **Cook Time:** 0 minutes | **Total Time:** 10 minutes + overnight | **Per Serving:** 2 servings

Ingredients:

- 1/4 cup chia seeds

- 1 cup unsweetened coconut milk

- 1 tablespoon maple syrup

- 1/2 cup diced mango

Instructions:

1. In a bowl or jar, combine chia seeds, coconut milk, and maple syrup.

2. Stir well to combine.

3. Cover and refrigerate overnight.

4. In the morning, give the chia pudding a good stir.

5. Top with diced mango before serving.

Nutritional Value: Calories: 200 | Protein: 4g | Carbohydrates: 24g | Fats: 10g | Sodium: 20mg | Potassium: 250mg | Fiber: 8g

Zucchini Fritters with Poached Eggs

Prep Time: 15 minutes | **Cook Time:** 10 minutes | **Total Time:** 25 minutes | **Per Serving:** 2 servings

Ingredients:

- 2 medium zucchinis, grated

- 1/4 cup flour

- 1 egg, beaten

- 2 green onions, chopped

- Salt and pepper, to taste

- 2 large eggs (for poaching)

- 2 tablespoons olive oil

Instructions:

1. Grate the zucchini and squeeze out excess moisture using a kitchen towel.

2. In a bowl, mix grated zucchini, flour, beaten egg, green onions, salt, and pepper.

3. Heat olive oil in a skillet over medium heat.

4. Drop spoonfuls of the zucchini mixture into the skillet and flatten with a spatula. Cook until golden brown on both sides, about 3-4 minutes per side.

5. Meanwhile, poach the eggs in simmering water.

6. Serve zucchini fritters topped with poached eggs.

Nutritional Value: Calories: 250 | Protein: 10g | Carbohydrates: 18g | Fats: 15g | Sodium: 150mg | Potassium: 450mg | Fiber: 3g

Oatmeal Pancakes with Blueberry Compote

Prep Time: 10 minutes | **Cook Time:** 20 minutes | **Total Time:** 30 minutes | **Per Serving:** 4 servings

Ingredients:

- 1 cup rolled oats

- 1 cup unsweetened almond milk

- 1 egg

- 1 tablespoon maple syrup

- 1 teaspoon baking powder

- 1/2 teaspoon vanilla extract

- Pinch of salt

- 1 cup fresh or frozen blueberries

- 1 tablespoon honey

Instructions:

1. In a blender, combine rolled oats, almond milk, egg, maple syrup, baking powder, vanilla extract, and salt. Blend until smooth.

2. Heat a non-stick skillet over medium heat. Pour batter onto the skillet, forming small pancakes.

3. Cook until bubbles form on the surface, then flip and cook until golden brown.

4. Meanwhile, in a small saucepan, combine blueberries and honey. Cook over medium heat until the blueberries break down and the mixture thickens.

5. Serve pancakes topped with blueberry compote.

Nutritional Value: Calories: 300 | Protein: 8g | Carbohydrates: 50g | Fats: 6g | Sodium: 200mg | Potassium: 200mg | Fiber: 7g

Lunch

Grilled Chicken Salad with Mixed Greens and Strawberries

Prep Time: 15 minutes | **Cook Time:** 10 minutes | **Total Time:** 25 minutes | **Per Serving:** 4 servings

Ingredients:

- 2 boneless, skinless chicken breasts
- 6 cups mixed greens
- 1 cup strawberries, sliced
- 1/4 cup sliced almonds
- 1/4 cup crumbled feta cheese (optional)
- 2 tablespoons balsamic vinegar
- 1 tablespoon extra virgin olive oil
- Salt and pepper, to taste

Instructions:

1. Preheat the grill to medium-high heat.
2. Season the chicken breasts with salt and pepper.
3. Grill the chicken for about 5-6 minutes on each side, or until fully cooked. Remove from grill and let rest.
4. In a large bowl, combine mixed greens, sliced strawberries, and sliced almonds.
5. In a small bowl, whisk together balsamic vinegar, olive oil, salt, and pepper.
6. Slice the grilled chicken breasts and add to the salad.
7. Drizzle the dressing over the salad and toss to combine.
8. Top with crumbled feta cheese if desired and serve immediately.

Nutritional Value: Calories: 350 | Protein: 30g | Carbohydrates: 15g | Fats: 18g | Sodium: 200mg | Potassium: 450mg | Fiber: 4g

Tuna Salad Stuffed Tomatoes

Prep Time: 15 minutes | **Cook Time:** 0 minutes | **Total Time:** 15 minutes | **Per Serving:** 4 servings

Ingredients:

- 4 large tomatoes
- 2 cans (5 ounces each) of tuna, drained
- 1/4 cup plain Greek yogurt
- 1/4 cup diced celery
- 1/4 cup diced red onion
- 1 tablespoon lemon juice
- 1 tablespoon fresh dill, chopped
- Salt and pepper, to taste

Instructions:

1. Cut the tops off the tomatoes and scoop out the insides.
2. In a bowl, combine tuna, Greek yogurt, celery, red onion, lemon juice, dill, salt, and pepper.
3. Stuff the hollowed-out tomatoes with the tuna mixture.
4. Serve immediately or chill until ready to serve.

Nutritional Value: Calories: 150 | Protein: 20g | Carbohydrates: 10g | Fats: 4g | Sodium: 200mg | Potassium: 350mg | Fiber: 2g

Lentil and Vegetable Soup with Whole Grain Crackers

Prep Time: 15 minutes | **Cook Time:** 30 minutes | **Total Time:** 45 minutes | **Per Serving:** 4 servings

Ingredients:

- 1 cup dried lentils, rinsed
- 1 carrot, diced
- 1 celery stalk, diced
- 1 onion, diced
- 2 cloves garlic, minced
- 6 cups vegetable broth
- 1 can (14.5 ounces) diced tomatoes
- 1 teaspoon cumin
- 1 teaspoon thyme
- Salt and pepper, to taste
- 1 cup spinach, chopped
- Whole grain crackers, for serving

Instructions:

1. In a large pot, heat a tablespoon of olive oil over medium heat.
2. Add diced carrot, celery, and onion, and sauté until softened.
3. Add minced garlic and cook for another minute.
4. Stir in lentils, vegetable broth, diced tomatoes, cumin, thyme, salt, and pepper.
5. Bring to a boil, then reduce heat and simmer for about 30 minutes, or until lentils are tender.
6. Stir in chopped spinach and cook until wilted.
7. Serve hot with whole-grain crackers on the side.

Nutritional Value: Calories: 250 | Protein: 12g | Carbohydrates: 40g | Fats: 3g | Sodium: 350mg | Potassium: 500mg | Fiber: 12g

Quinoa and Roasted Vegetable Bowl with Tahini Dressing

Prep Time: 15 minutes | **Cook Time:** 25 minutes | **Total Time:** 40 minutes | **Per Serving:** 4 servings

Ingredients:

- 1 cup quinoa, rinsed
- 2 cups water
- 1 zucchini, diced
- 1 bell pepper, diced
- 1 red onion, diced
- 1 cup cherry tomatoes, halved
- 2 tablespoons olive oil
- Salt and pepper, to taste
- 1/4 cup tahini
- 2 tablespoons lemon juice
- 1 clove garlic, minced
- Water to thin dressing

Instructions:

1. Preheat oven to 400°F (200°C).

2. On a baking sheet, toss zucchini, bell pepper, red onion, and cherry tomatoes with olive oil, salt, and pepper. Roast for 20-25 minutes.

3. Meanwhile, in a saucepan, combine quinoa and water. Bring to a boil, then reduce heat and simmer until water is absorbed and quinoa is tender, about 15 minutes.

4. In a small bowl, whisk together tahini, lemon juice, minced garlic, and enough water to reach a drizzling consistency. Season with salt.

5. To assemble, divide cooked quinoa into bowls, top with roasted vegetables, and drizzle with tahini dressing.

6. Serve immediately.

Nutritional Value: Calories: 350 | Protein: 10g | Carbohydrates: 40g | Fats: 16g | Sodium: 200mg | Potassium: 400mg | Fiber: 8g

Grilled Salmon and Asparagus Foil Packets

Prep Time: 10 minutes | **Cook Time:** 20 minutes | **Total Time:** 30 minutes | **Per Serving:** 4 servings

Ingredients:

- 4 salmon fillets

- 1 bunch asparagus, trimmed

- 2 tablespoons olive oil

- 1 lemon, thinly sliced

- Salt and pepper, to taste

- Fresh dill, for garnish

Instructions:

1. Preheat the grill to medium-high heat.

2. Place each salmon fillet on a piece of aluminum foil.

3. Divide asparagus among the foil packets, placing them next to the salmon.

4. Drizzle olive oil over salmon and asparagus, and season with salt and pepper.

5. Top each salmon fillet with lemon slices.

6. Fold the foil over the salmon and asparagus to create a packet.

7. Grill for 15-20 minutes, or until salmon is cooked through and asparagus is tender.

8. Carefully open the foil packets and garnish with fresh dill before serving.

Nutritional Value: Calories: 300 | Protein: 28g | Carbohydrates: 8g | Fats: 18g | Sodium: 180mg | Potassium: 600mg | Fiber: 3g

Chickpea and Cucumber Salad with Lemon Vinaigrette

Prep Time: 15 minutes | **Cook Time:** 0 minutes | **Total Time:** 15 minutes | **Per Serving:** 4 servings

Ingredients:

- 2 cans (15 ounces each) chickpeas, drained and rinsed

- 1 cucumber, diced

- 1/2 red onion, thinly sliced

- 1/4 cup fresh parsley, chopped

- 1/4 cup lemon juice

- 2 tablespoons olive oil

- 1 clove garlic, minced

- Salt and pepper, to taste

Instructions:

1. In a large bowl, combine chickpeas, cucumber, red onion, and parsley.

2. In a small bowl, whisk together lemon juice, olive oil, garlic, salt, and pepper.

3. Pour the dressing over the chickpea mixture and toss until well combined.

4. Serve immediately or refrigerate until ready to serve.

Nutritional Value: Calories: 200 | Protein: 7g | Carbohydrates: 28g | Fats: 7g | Sodium: 180mg | Potassium: 350mg | Fiber: 6g

Turkey and Avocado Lettuce Wraps

Prep Time: 10 minutes | **Cook Time:** 0 minutes | **Total Time:** 10 minutes | **Per Serving:** 4 servings

Ingredients:

- 1 pound cooked turkey breast, thinly sliced

- 1 avocado, sliced

- 1 head of romaine lettuce, leaves separated

- 1/4 cup hummus

- 1/2 cup shredded carrots

- Salt and pepper, to taste

Instructions:

1. Lay out the lettuce leaves on a plate.

2. Spread a small amount of hummus on each lettuce leaf.

3. Top with slices of turkey, avocado, and shredded carrots.

4. Season with salt and pepper.

5. Roll up the lettuce leaves and serve immediately.

Nutritional Value: Calories: 180 | Protein: 20g | Carbohydrates: 8g | Fats: 8g | Sodium: 250mg | Potassium: 400mg | Fiber: 4g

Roasted Butternut Squash and Kale Salad with Pumpkin Seeds

Prep Time: 15 minutes | **Cook Time:** 25 minutes | **Total Time:** 40 minutes | **Per Serving:** 4 servings

Ingredients:

- 1 small butternut squash, peeled and cubed

- 2 tablespoons olive oil

- Salt and pepper, to taste

- 6 cups kale, chopped

- 1/4 cup pumpkin seeds

- 2 tablespoons balsamic vinegar

- 1 tablespoon honey

Instructions:

1. Preheat oven to 400°F (200°C).

2. Toss the butternut squash cubes with olive oil, salt, and pepper. Spread on a baking sheet and roast for 25 minutes, or until tender.

3. In a large bowl, combine the chopped kale and roasted butternut squash.

4. In a small bowl, whisk together balsamic vinegar and honey. Pour over the salad and toss to combine.

5. Sprinkle with pumpkin seeds and serve immediately.

Nutritional Value: Calories: 220 | Protein: 5g | Carbohydrates: 30g | Fats: 10g | Sodium: 150mg | Potassium: 500mg | Fiber: 7g

Baked Cod with Roasted Brussels Sprouts and Garlic

Prep Time: 10 minutes | **Cook Time:** 25 minutes | **Total Time:** 35 minutes | **Per Serving:** 4 servings

Ingredients:

- 4 cod fillets
- 1 pound Brussels sprouts, halved
- 4 cloves garlic, minced
- 3 tablespoons olive oil
- Salt and pepper, to taste
- Lemon wedges, for serving

Instructions:

1. Preheat oven to 400°F (200°C).
2. Toss Brussels sprouts and garlic with 2 tablespoons olive oil, salt, and pepper. Spread on a baking sheet and roast for 15 minutes.
3. Place cod fillets on another baking sheet. Drizzle with remaining olive oil, and season with salt and pepper.
4. After the Brussels sprouts have roasted for 15 minutes, add the cod to the oven and roast for an additional 10 minutes, or until the cod is cooked through and the Brussels sprouts are tender.
5. Serve the baked cod with roasted Brussels sprouts and lemon wedges.

Nutritional Value: Calories: 250 | Protein: 30g | Carbohydrates: 10g | Fats: 10g | Sodium: 150mg | Potassium: 600mg | Fiber: 4g

Tofu and Vegetable Stir-Fry over Brown Rice

Prep Time: 15 minutes | **Cook Time:** 15 minutes | **Total Time:** 30 minutes | **Per Serving:** 4 servings

Ingredients:

- 1 block (14 ounces) of firm tofu, pressed and cubed

- 2 tablespoons soy sauce (low sodium)

- 1 tablespoon sesame oil

- 2 cloves garlic, minced

- 1 bell pepper, sliced

- 1 carrot, julienned

- 1 cup broccoli florets

- 2 tablespoons hoisin sauce

- 2 cups cooked brown rice

- Green onions, sliced, for garnish

Instructions:

1. In a bowl, toss cubed tofu with soy sauce and sesame oil.

2. Heat a non-stick skillet over medium heat. Add tofu and cook until golden brown. Remove and set aside.

3. In the same skillet, add garlic, bell pepper, carrot, and broccoli. Stir-fry until vegetables are tender.

4. Return tofu to the skillet and add hoisin sauce. Stir until everything is well coated and heated through.

5. Serve stir-fry over cooked brown rice, garnished with sliced green onions.

Nutritional Value: Calories: 350 | Protein: 15g | Carbohydrates: 50g | Fats: 10g | Sodium: 400mg | Potassium: 500mg | Fiber: 6g

Dinner

Grilled Chicken Kebabs with Bell Peppers and Zucchini

Prep Time: 20 minutes | **Cook Time:** 10 minutes | **Total Time:** 30 minutes | **Per Serving:** 4 servings

Ingredients:

- 2 boneless, skinless chicken breasts, cut into cubes
- 1 red bell pepper, cut into chunks
- 1 yellow bell pepper, cut into chunks
- 1 zucchini, sliced
- 2 tablespoons olive oil
- 2 tablespoons lemon juice
- 2 cloves garlic, minced
- 1 teaspoon dried oregano
- Salt and pepper, to taste
- Wooden skewers, soaked in water

Instructions:

1. In a bowl, whisk together olive oil, lemon juice, minced garlic, dried oregano, salt, and pepper.

2. Thread chicken cubes, bell pepper chunks, and zucchini slices onto skewers.

3. Brush the skewers with the marinade.

4. Preheat the grill to medium-high heat.

5. Grill the kebabs for 5 minutes on each side, or until the chicken is cooked through and the vegetables are tender.

6. Serve immediately.

Nutritional Value: Calories: 250 | Protein: 25g | Carbohydrates: 10g | Fats: 12g | Sodium: 150mg | Potassium: 350mg | Phosphorus: 200mg | Fiber: 3g

Baked Salmon with Roasted Sweet Potatoes and Green Beans

Prep Time: 15 minutes | **Cook Time:** 25 minutes | **Total Time:** 40 minutes | **Per Serving:** 4 servings

Ingredients:

- 4 salmon fillets
- 2 sweet potatoes, peeled and cubed
- 1 pound green beans, trimmed
- 2 tablespoons olive oil
- 1 tablespoon lemon juice
- 2 cloves garlic, minced
- Salt and pepper, to taste
- Fresh dill, for garnish

Instructions:

1. Preheat oven to 400°F (200°C).
2. Place sweet potato cubes and green beans on a baking sheet.
3. Drizzle with olive oil, lemon juice, minced garlic, salt, and pepper. Toss to coat.
4. Push vegetables to the sides of the baking sheet and place salmon fillets in the center.
5. Season salmon with salt and pepper.
6. Bake for 20-25 minutes, or until salmon is cooked through and vegetables are tender.
7. Garnish with fresh dill before serving.

Nutritional Value: Calories: 300 | Protein: 25g | Carbohydrates: 20g | Fats: 12g | Sodium: 150mg | Potassium: 500mg | Phosphorus: 250mg | Fiber: 5g

Lentil and Vegetable Curry over Cauliflower Rice

Prep Time: 15 minutes | **Cook Time:** 25 minutes | **Total Time:** 40 minutes | **Per Serving:** 4 servings

Ingredients:

- 1 cup dry lentils, rinsed
- 1 tablespoon olive oil
- 1 onion, diced
- 2 cloves garlic, minced
- 1 tablespoon curry powder
- 1 teaspoon ground cumin
- 1 teaspoon ground coriander
- 1/2 teaspoon ground turmeric
- 1/4 teaspoon cayenne pepper (optional)
- 1 can (14.5 ounces) diced tomatoes
- 1 can (13.5 ounces) coconut milk
- 2 cups cauliflower rice
- Salt and pepper, to taste
- Fresh cilantro, for garnish

Instructions:

1. In a large skillet, heat olive oil over medium heat.
2. Add diced onion and minced garlic, and sauté until softened.
3. Stir in curry powder, ground cumin, ground coriander, ground turmeric, and cayenne pepper (if using). Cook for another minute.
4. Add diced tomatoes (with juices), coconut milk, and dry lentils. Bring to a simmer and cook for about 20-25 minutes, or until lentils are tender.
5. While the curry is cooking, steam cauliflower rice until tender.
6. Season the lentil curry with salt and pepper to taste.
7. Serve the lentil curry over cauliflower rice, garnished with fresh cilantro.

Nutritional Value: Calories: 300 | Protein: 15g | Carbohydrates: 30g | Fats: 15g | Sodium: 200mg | Potassium: 400mg | Phosphorus: 200mg | Fiber: 10g

Grilled Pork Tenderloin with Roasted Apples and Onions

Prep Time: 15 minutes | **Cook Time:** 25 minutes | **Total Time:** 40 minutes | **Per Serving:** 4 servings

Ingredients:

- 1 pork tenderloin (about 1 pound)
- 2 apples, cored and sliced
- 1 red onion, sliced
- 2 tablespoons olive oil
- 2 tablespoons balsamic vinegar
- 1 tablespoon honey
- 1 teaspoon dried thyme
- Salt and pepper, to taste

Instructions:

1. Preheat the grill to medium-high heat.
2. Season pork tenderloin with salt, pepper, and dried thyme.
3. In a bowl, whisk together olive oil, balsamic vinegar, and honey.
4. Toss sliced apples and onions with half of the olive oil mixture.
5. Grill pork tenderloin for about 20-25 minutes, turning occasionally, until cooked through.
6. Meanwhile, roast the apple and onion mixture in the oven at 400°F (200°C) for 15-20 minutes, or until tender and caramelized.
7. Serve grilled pork tenderloin with roasted apples and onions.

Nutritional Value: Calories: 250 | Protein: 25g | Carbohydrates: 20g | Fats: 10g | Sodium: 150mg | Potassium: 400mg | Phosphorus: 200mg | Fiber: 4g

Quinoa and Black Bean Stuffed Bell Peppers

Prep Time: 15 minutes | **Cook Time:** 30 minutes | **Total Time:** 45 minutes | **Per Serving:** 4 servings

Ingredients:

- 4 bell peppers, halved and seeded
- 1 cup quinoa, cooked
- 1 can (15 ounces) black beans, drained and rinsed
- 1 cup corn kernels
- 1/2 cup diced tomatoes
- 1/2 cup diced red onion
- 1/4 cup chopped fresh cilantro
- 1 teaspoon ground cumin
- 1/2 teaspoon chili powder
- Salt and pepper, to taste
- 1/2 cup shredded low-fat cheese (optional)

Instructions:

1. Preheat oven to 375°F (190°C).

2. In a large bowl, combine cooked quinoa, black beans, corn kernels, diced tomatoes, diced red onion, chopped cilantro, ground cumin, chili powder, salt, and pepper.

3. Spoon the quinoa and black bean mixture into the halved bell peppers.

4. Place stuffed bell peppers in a baking dish. Cover with foil and bake for 25 minutes or until peppers are tender. 5. If using cheese, remove the foil and sprinkle shredded cheese over the stuffed peppers.

5. Return to the oven and bake for an additional 5 minutes, or until the cheese is melted and bubbly.

6. Remove from the oven and let cool slightly before serving.

Nutritional Value: Calories: 300 | Protein: 15g | Carbohydrates: 50g | Fats: 5g | Sodium: 200mg | Potassium: 400mg | Phosphorus: 150mg | Fiber: 12g

Baked Tilapia with Roasted Broccoli and Garlic

Prep Time: 10 minutes | **Cook Time:** 20 minutes | **Total Time:** 30 minutes | **Per Serving:** 4 servings

Ingredients:

- 4 tilapia fillets

- 1 pound broccoli florets

- 4 cloves garlic, minced

- 2 tablespoons olive oil

- Salt and pepper, to taste

- Lemon wedges, for serving

Instructions:

1. Preheat oven to 400°F (200°C).

2. Place tilapia fillets on a baking sheet lined with parchment paper.

3. In a bowl, toss broccoli florets with minced garlic, olive oil, salt, and pepper.

4. Spread the broccoli mixture around the tilapia fillets on the baking sheet.

5. Bake for 15-20 minutes, or until tilapia is cooked through and flakes easily with a fork.

6. Serve baked tilapia with roasted broccoli and garlic, accompanied by lemon wedges.

Nutritional Value: Calories: 200 | Protein: 25g | Carbohydrates: 15g | Fats: 8g | Sodium: 150mg | Potassium: 450mg | Phosphorus: 200mg | Fiber: 6g

Tofu and Vegetable Stir-Fry with Brown Rice Noodles

Prep Time: 15 minutes | **Cook Time:** 15 minutes | **Total Time:** 30 minutes | **Per Serving:** 4 servings

Ingredients:

- 1 block (14 ounces) of firm tofu, cubed
- 8 ounces brown rice noodles
- 2 tablespoons soy sauce (low sodium)
- 1 tablespoon sesame oil
- 1 tablespoon rice vinegar
- 1 tablespoon honey
- 2 cloves garlic, minced
- 1 tablespoon grated ginger
- 1 bell pepper, sliced
- 1 carrot, julienned
- 1 cup broccoli florets
- 2 green onions, sliced
- Sesame seeds, for garnish

Instructions:

1. Cook brown rice noodles according to package instructions. Drain and set aside.

2. In a small bowl, whisk together soy sauce, sesame oil, rice vinegar, honey, minced garlic, and grated ginger to make the sauce.

3. Heat a large skillet or wok over medium-high heat. Add tofu cubes and stir-fry until golden brown.

4. Add sliced bell pepper, julienned carrot, and broccoli florets to the skillet. Stir-fry for 3-4 minutes, or until vegetables are tender-crisp.

5. Add cooked brown rice noodles and sauce to the skillet. Toss everything together until well combined and heated through.

6. Serve tofu and vegetable stir-fry over brown rice noodles, garnished with sliced green onions and sesame seeds.

Nutritional Value: Calories: 300 | Protein: 15g | Carbohydrates: 40g | Fats: 10g | Sodium: 250mg | Potassium: 400mg | Phosphorus: 200mg | Fiber: 6g

Grilled Shrimp Skewers with Mango Salsa and Cauliflower Rice

Prep Time: 20 minutes | **Cook Time:** 10 minutes | **Total Time:** 30 minutes | **Per Serving:** 4 servings

Ingredients:

- 1 pound large shrimp, peeled and deveined
- 1 mango, diced
- 1/2 red onion, diced
- 1 jalapeño pepper, seeded and minced
- 1/4 cup chopped fresh cilantro
- 2 tablespoons lime juice
- Salt and pepper, to taste
- 1 head cauliflower, riced
- Wooden skewers, soaked in water

Instructions:

1. Preheat the grill to medium-high heat.
2. Thread shrimp onto skewers.
3. In a bowl, combine diced mango, diced red onion, minced jalapeño pepper, chopped cilantro, lime juice, salt, and pepper to make the salsa. Set aside.
4. Grill shrimp skewers for 2-3 minutes on each side, or until shrimp are pink and opaque.
5. Meanwhile, steam cauliflower rice until tender.
6. Serve grilled shrimp skewers over cauliflower rice, topped with mango salsa.

Nutritional Value: Calories: 200 | Protein: 25g | Carbohydrates: 15g | Fats: 5g | Sodium: 200mg | Potassium: 350mg | Phosphorus: 150mg | Fiber: 5g

Baked Chicken Parmesan with Zucchini Noodles

Prep Time: 20 minutes | **Cook Time:** 25 minutes | **Total Time:** 45 minutes | **Per Serving:** 4 servings

Ingredients:

- 4 boneless, skinless chicken breasts
- 1 cup marinara sauce (low sodium)
- 1/2 cup shredded mozzarella cheese (low sodium)
- 1/4 cup grated Parmesan cheese
- 2 medium zucchinis
- 1 tablespoon olive oil
- Salt and pepper, to taste
- Fresh basil leaves, for garnish

Instructions:

1. Preheat oven to 400°F (200°C).
2. Season chicken breasts with salt and pepper.
3. Place chicken breasts on a baking sheet lined with parchment paper.
4. Spread marinara sauce over each chicken breast.
5. Sprinkle shredded mozzarella cheese and grated Parmesan cheese over the marinara sauce.
6. Bake for 20-25 minutes, or until chicken is cooked through and cheese is melted and bubbly.
7. While the chicken is baking, use a spiralizer to make zucchini noodles.
8. Heat olive oil in a skillet over medium heat. Add zucchini noodles and sauté for 2-3 minutes, or until tender.
9. Serve baked chicken Parmesan over zucchini noodles, garnished with fresh basil leaves.

Nutritional Value: Calories: 300 | Protein: 35g | Carbohydrates: 10g | Fats: 12g | Sodium: 250mg | Potassium: 400mg | Phosphorus: 250mg | Fiber: 3g

Lentil and Sweet Potato Shepherd's Pie

Prep Time: 20 minutes | **Cook Time:** 40 minutes | **Total Time:** 1 hour | **Per Serving:** 4 servings

Ingredients:

- 1 cup dry green or brown lentils, rinsed
- 2 cups vegetable broth (low sodium)
- 2 tablespoons olive oil
- 1 onion, chopped
- 2 cloves garlic, minced
- 2 carrots, diced
- 2 stalks celery, diced
- 1 teaspoon dried thyme
- 1 teaspoon dried rosemary
- 2 cups sweet potatoes, peeled and cubed
- 1/4 cup unsweetened almond milk
- Salt and pepper, to taste

Instructions:

1. In a medium saucepan, combine rinsed lentils and vegetable broth. Bring to a boil, then reduce heat and simmer for 20-25 minutes, or until lentils are tender.
2. Preheat oven to 375°F (190°C).
3. Heat olive oil in a large skillet over medium heat. Add chopped onion and minced garlic, and sauté until softened.
4. Add diced carrots and celery to the skillet, and cook for another 5 minutes.
5. Stir in dried thyme and dried rosemary.
6. Add cooked lentils to the skillet and mix well. Season with salt and pepper to taste.

7. In a separate pot, boil sweet potatoes until tender. Drain and mash with unsweetened almond milk until smooth.

8. Transfer the lentil mixture to a baking dish and spread mashed sweet potatoes over the top.

9. Bake in the preheated oven for 20-25 minutes, or until the top is golden brown.

10. Serve hot.

Nutritional Value: Calories: 300 | Protein: 15g | Carbohydrates: 45g | Fats: 8g | Sodium: 200mg | Potassium: 500mg | Phosphorus: 250mg | Fiber: 12g

Soup

Chicken and Vegetable Soup with Whole Grain Crackers

Prep Time: 15 minutes | **Cook Time:** 30 minutes | **Total Time:** 45 minutes | **Per Serving:** 4 servings

Ingredients:

- 2 boneless, skinless chicken breasts
- 6 cups low-sodium chicken broth
- 2 carrots, diced
- 2 celery stalks, diced
- 1 onion, diced
- 2 cloves garlic, minced
- 1 cup green beans, chopped
- 1 cup cabbage, shredded
- 1 bay leaf
- 1 teaspoon dried thyme
- Salt and pepper, to taste
- Whole grain crackers, for serving

Instructions:

1. In a large pot, combine chicken broth, diced carrots, diced celery, diced onion, minced garlic, bay leaf, and dried thyme.

2. Bring the broth to a boil, then reduce heat and simmer for 15 minutes.

3. Add chicken breasts to the pot and continue to simmer for another 15 minutes, or until the chicken is cooked through.

4. Remove chicken breasts from the pot and shred them with two forks. Return shredded chicken to the pot.

5. Add chopped green beans and shredded cabbage to the pot. Simmer for an additional 5 minutes.

6. Season the soup with salt and pepper to taste.

7. Serve hot with whole-grain crackers on the side.

Nutritional Value: Calories: 200 | Protein: 20g | Carbohydrates: 15g | Fats: 5g | Sodium: 200mg | Potassium: 250mg | Phosphorus: 150mg | Fiber: 5g

Butternut Squash Soup with Roasted Chickpeas

Prep Time: 15 minutes | **Cook Time:** 45 minutes | **Total Time:** 1 hour | **Per Serving:** 4 servings

Ingredients:

- 1 butternut squash, peeled, seeded, and cubed
- 1 onion, diced
- 2 cloves garlic, minced
- 4 cups low-sodium vegetable broth
- 1 teaspoon dried thyme
- 1/2 teaspoon ground cinnamon
- 1/4 teaspoon ground nutmeg
- Salt and pepper, to taste
- 1 can (15 ounces) chickpeas, drained and rinsed
- 1 tablespoon olive oil

Instructions:

1. Preheat oven to 400°F (200°C).

2. In a large pot, combine cubed butternut squash, diced onion, minced garlic, vegetable broth, dried thyme, ground cinnamon, and ground nutmeg.

3. Bring the mixture to a boil, then reduce heat and simmer for 30 minutes, or until squash is tender.

4. While the soup is cooking, toss chickpeas with olive oil, salt, and pepper. Spread on a baking sheet and roast in the preheated oven for 20-25 minutes or until crispy.

5. Once the squash is tender, use an immersion blender to puree the soup until smooth.

6. Season the soup with salt and pepper to taste.

7. Serve hot, topped with roasted chickpeas.

Nutritional Value: Calories: 250 | Protein: 10g | Carbohydrates: 40g | Fats: 5g | Sodium: 200mg | Potassium: 400mg | Phosphorus: 150mg | Fiber: 10g

Minestrone Soup with Spinach and Whole Grain Pasta

Prep Time: 15 minutes | **Cook Time:** 30 minutes | **Total Time:** 45 minutes | **Per Serving:** 4 servings

Ingredients:

- 1 tablespoon olive oil
- 1 onion, diced
- 2 carrots, diced
- 2 celery stalks, diced
- 2 cloves garlic, minced
- 6 cups low-sodium vegetable broth
- 1 can (15 ounces) diced tomatoes
- 1 can (15 ounces) kidney beans, drained and rinsed
- 1 cup whole-grain pasta
- 2 cups fresh spinach
- 1 teaspoon dried oregano
- 1 teaspoon dried basil
- Salt and pepper, to taste

Instructions:

1. In a large pot, heat olive oil over medium heat. Add diced onion, diced carrots, diced celery, and minced garlic. Sauté until vegetables are tender.

2. Add low-sodium vegetable broth, diced tomatoes (with juices), and drained kidney beans to the pot. Bring to a boil.

3. Stir in whole-grain pasta, dried oregano, and dried basil. Simmer for 10-12 minutes, or until pasta is al dente.

4. Add fresh spinach to the pot and cook for an additional 2-3 minutes, or until wilted.

5. Season the soup with salt and pepper to taste.

6. Serve hot.

Nutritional Value: Calories: 250 | Protein: 10g | Carbohydrates: 40g | Fats: 5g | Sodium: 200mg | Potassium: 300mg | Phosphorus: 150mg | Fiber: 8g

Lentil and Kale Soup with Whole Grain Bread

Prep Time: 15 minutes | **Cook Time:** 45 minutes | **Total Time:** 1 hour | **Per Serving:** 4 servings

Ingredients:

- 1 cup dry green or brown lentils, rinsed
- 6 cups low-sodium vegetable broth
- 1 onion, diced
- 2 cloves garlic, minced
- 2 carrots, diced
- 2 celery stalks, diced
- 1 teaspoon dried thyme
- 1 teaspoon dried rosemary
- 2 cups chopped kale
- Salt and pepper, to taste
- Whole grain bread, for serving

Instructions:

1. In a large pot, combine rinsed lentils, low-sodium vegetable broth, diced onion, minced garlic, diced carrots, diced celery, dried thyme, and dried rosemary.
2. Bring the mixture to a boil, then reduce heat and simmer for 30-35 minutes, or until lentils are tender.
3. Add chopped kale to the pot and cook for an additional 5 minutes, or until kale is wilted.
4. Season the soup with salt and pepper to taste.
5. Serve hot with whole grain bread on the side.

Nutritional Value: Calories: 250 | Protein: 15g | Carbohydrates: 40g | Fats: 5g | Sodium: 200mg | Potassium: 300mg | Phosphorus: 150mg | Fiber: 10g

Roasted Tomato and Basil Soup with Grilled Cheese Croutons

Prep Time: 15 minutes | **Cook Time:** 1 hour | **Total Time:** 1 hour 15 minutes | **Per Serving:** 4 servings

Ingredients:

- 1 1/2 pounds plum tomatoes, halved

- 1 onion, quartered

- 4 cloves garlic, peeled

- 2 tablespoons olive oil

- 1 teaspoon dried oregano

- 1/2 teaspoon dried thyme

- Salt and pepper, to taste

- 4 cups low-sodium vegetable broth

- 1/4 cup fresh basil leaves, plus more for garnish

- 4 slices whole grain bread

- 1/2 cup shredded mozzarella cheese (low sodium)

Instructions:

1. Preheat oven to 400°F (200°C).

2. Place halved tomatoes, quartered onion, and peeled garlic cloves on a baking sheet. Drizzle with olive oil and sprinkle with dried oregano, dried thyme, salt, and pepper. Toss to coat.

3. Roast in the preheated oven for 45-50 minutes, or until vegetables are soft and caramelized.

4. Transfer roasted vegetables to a large pot. Add low-sodium vegetable broth and fresh basil leaves.

5. Use an immersion blender to puree the soup until smooth. Alternatively, you can transfer the mixture to a blender and blend until smooth, then return to the pot.

6. Season the soup with salt and pepper to taste.

7. Heat a non-stick skillet over medium heat. Place a slice of whole-grain bread in the skillet and top with shredded mozzarella cheese. Place another slice of bread on top to make a sandwich.

8. Cook until the bread is golden brown and the cheese is melted. Repeat with the remaining bread slices.

9. Cut the grilled cheese sandwiches into bite-sized pieces to make croutons.

10. Ladle the roasted tomato and basil soup into bowls and garnish with grilled cheese croutons and fresh basil leaves.

Nutritional Value: Calories: 250 | Protein: 10g | Carbohydrates: 30g | Fats: 10g | Sodium: 200mg | Potassium: 350mg | Phosphorus: 150mg | Fiber: 6g

Chicken and Wild Rice Soup with Celery and Carrots

Prep Time: 15 minutes | **Cook Time:** 45 minutes | **Total Time:** 1 hour | **Per Serving:** 4 servings

Ingredients:

- 2 boneless, skinless chicken breasts

- 1/2 cup wild rice

- 6 cups low-sodium chicken broth

- 2 carrots, diced

- 2 celery stalks, diced

- 1 onion, diced

- 2 cloves garlic, minced

- 1 teaspoon dried thyme

- Salt and pepper, to taste

Instructions:

1. In a large pot, combine chicken broth, diced carrots, diced celery, diced onion, minced garlic, dried thyme, and wild rice.

2. Bring the mixture to a boil, then reduce heat and simmer for 30-35 minutes, or until rice is tender.

3. Meanwhile, cook chicken breasts in a separate pot of boiling water for 15-20 minutes, or until cooked through. Remove from water and shred with two forks.

4. Add shredded chicken to the soup and simmer for an additional 10 minutes.

5. Season the soup with salt and pepper to taste.

6. Serve hot.

Nutritional Value: Calories: 250 | Protein: 20g | Carbohydrates: 30g | Fats: 5g | Sodium: 200mg | Potassium: 300mg | Phosphorus: 150mg | Fiber: 5g

Vegetable and Barley Soup with Whole Grain Rolls

Prep Time: 15 minutes | **Cook Time:** 45 minutes | **Total Time:** 1 hour | **Per Serving:** 4 servings

Ingredients:

- 1/2 cup pearl barley

- 6 cups low-sodium vegetable broth

- 2 carrots, diced

- 2 celery stalks, diced

- 1 onion, diced

- 2 cloves garlic, minced

- 1 cup green beans, chopped

- 1 cup cabbage, shredded

- 1 teaspoon dried thyme

- Salt and pepper, to taste

- Whole grain rolls, for serving

Instructions:

1. In a large pot, combine vegetable broth, pearl barley, diced carrots, diced celery, diced onion, minced garlic, chopped green beans, shredded cabbage, and dried thyme.

2. Bring the mixture to a boil, then reduce heat and simmer for 30-35 minutes, or until the barley is tender.

3. Season the soup with salt and pepper to taste.

4. Serve hot with whole grain rolls on the side.

Nutritional Value: Calories: 200 | Protein: 5g | Carbohydrates: 40g | Fats: 2g | Sodium: 150mg | Potassium: 250mg | Phosphorus: 100mg | Fiber: 8g

Creamy Cauliflower Soup with Roasted Garlic

Prep Time: 10 minutes | **Cook Time:** 40 minutes | **Total Time:** 50 minutes | **Per Serving:** 4 servings

Ingredients:

- 1 head cauliflower, chopped

- 1 onion, diced

- 4 cloves garlic, peeled

- 4 cups low-sodium vegetable broth

- 1/2 cup unsweetened almond milk

- Salt and pepper, to taste

Instructions:

1. Preheat oven to 400°F (200°C).

2. Place chopped cauliflower, diced onion, and peeled garlic cloves on a baking sheet. Drizzle with olive oil and season with salt and pepper.

3. Roast in the preheated oven for 25-30 minutes, or until cauliflower is tender and caramelized.

4. Transfer roasted cauliflower, onion, and garlic to a large pot. Add low-sodium vegetable broth.

5. Bring the mixture to a boil, then reduce heat and simmer for 10-15 minutes.

6. Use an immersion blender to puree the soup until smooth.

7. Stir in unsweetened almond milk and heat through.

8. Season the soup with salt and pepper to taste.

9. Serve hot.

Nutritional Value: Calories: 150 | Protein: 5g | Carbohydrates: 20g | Fats: 6g | Sodium: 200mg | Potassium: 300mg | Phosphorus: 100mg | Fiber: 5g

Turkey and Vegetable Noodle Soup with Whole Grain Noodles

Prep Time: 15 minutes | **Cook Time:** 30 minutes | **Total Time:** 45 minutes | **Per Serving:** 4 servings

Ingredients:

- 8 cups low-sodium chicken broth
- 2 cups cooked turkey breast, shredded
- 2 carrots, diced
- 2 celery stalks, diced
- 1 onion, diced
- 2 cloves garlic, minced
- 2 cups whole grain noodles
- 1 teaspoon dried thyme
- Salt and pepper, to taste

Instructions:

1. In a large pot, combine low-sodium chicken broth, shredded turkey breast, diced carrots, diced celery, diced onion, minced garlic, whole grain noodles, and dried thyme.

2. Bring the mixture to a boil, then reduce heat and simmer for 20-25 minutes, or until noodles are tender.

3. Season the soup with salt and pepper to taste.

4. Serve hot.

Nutritional Value: Calories: 300 | Protein: 25g | Carbohydrates: 30g | Fats: 8g | Sodium: 200mg | Potassium: 250mg | Phosphorus: 150mg | Fiber: 5g

Broccoli and Cheddar Soup with Whole Grain Crackers

Prep Time: 10 minutes | **Cook Time:** 30 minutes | **Total Time:** 40 minutes | **Per Serving:** 4 servings

Ingredients:

- 2 cups broccoli florets
- 1 onion, diced
- 2 cloves garlic, minced
- 4 cups low-sodium vegetable broth
- 1/2 cup unsweetened almond milk
- 1 cup shredded low-sodium cheddar cheese
- Salt and pepper, to taste
- Whole grain crackers, for serving

Instructions:

1. In a large pot, combine broccoli florets, diced onion, minced garlic, and low-sodium vegetable broth.
2. Bring the mixture to a boil, then reduce heat and simmer for 15-20 minutes, or until broccoli is tender.
3. Use an immersion blender to puree the soup until smooth.
4. Stir in unsweetened almond milk and shredded low-sodium cheddar cheese until cheese is melted.
5. Season the soup with salt and pepper to taste.
6. Serve hot with whole-grain crackers on the side.

Nutritional Value: Calories: 250 | Protein: 15g | Carbohydrates: 20g | Fats: 10g | Sodium: 200mg | Potassium: 300mg | Phosphorus: 150mg | Fiber: 5g

Vegetarian Options

Lentil and Sweet Potato Curry with Cauliflower Rice

Prep Time: 15 minutes | **Cook Time:** 30 minutes | **Total Time:** 45 minutes | **Per Serving:** 4 servings

Ingredients:

- 1 cup dry green or brown lentils, rinsed

- 2 cups low-sodium vegetable broth

- 2 sweet potatoes, peeled and diced

- 1 onion, diced

- 2 cloves garlic, minced

- 1 tablespoon curry powder

- 1 teaspoon ground turmeric

- 1 teaspoon ground cumin

- 1/2 teaspoon ground ginger

- 1 can (14 ounces) low-sodium diced tomatoes

- 1 can (14 ounces) coconut milk

- Salt and pepper, to taste

- 1 head cauliflower, riced

- Fresh cilantro, for garnish

Instructions:

1. In a large pot, combine rinsed lentils and low-sodium vegetable broth. Bring to a boil, then reduce heat and simmer for 20-25 minutes, or until lentils are tender.

2. In a separate pot, steam diced sweet potatoes until tender, about 10-15 minutes. Set aside.

3. In a large skillet, sauté diced onion and minced garlic until softened.

4. Add curry powder, ground turmeric, ground cumin, and ground ginger to the skillet. Cook for 1-2 minutes, until fragrant.

5. Stir in low-sodium diced tomatoes (with juices) and coconut milk. Bring to a simmer.

6. Add cooked lentils and diced sweet potatoes to the skillet. Simmer for 5-10 minutes to allow flavors to blend.

7. Season the curry with salt and pepper to taste.

8. Serve hot over cauliflower rice, garnished with fresh cilantro.

Nutritional Value: Calories: 300 | Protein: 10g | Carbohydrates: 40g | Fats: 10g | Sodium: 150mg | Potassium: 400mg | Phosphorus: 200mg | Fiber: 12g

Quinoa and Black Bean Stuffed Portobello Mushrooms

Prep Time: 15 minutes | **Cook Time:** 25 minutes | **Total Time:** 40 minutes | **Per Serving:** 4 servings

Ingredients:

- 4 large portobello mushrooms

- 1 cup cooked quinoa

- 1 can (15 ounces) low-sodium black beans, drained and rinsed

- 1/2 red bell pepper, diced

- 1/2 green bell pepper, diced

- 1/2 onion, diced

- 2 cloves garlic, minced

- 1 teaspoon ground cumin

- 1/2 teaspoon chili powder

- Salt and pepper, to taste

- Fresh cilantro, for garnish

Instructions:

1. Preheat oven to 375°F (190°C).

2. Remove stems from portobello mushrooms and gently scrape out the gills using a spoon.

3. In a large bowl, combine cooked quinoa, low-sodium black beans, diced red bell pepper, diced green bell pepper, diced onion, minced garlic, ground cumin, and chili powder. Season with salt and pepper to taste.

4. Stuff each portobello mushroom with the quinoa and black bean mixture.

5. Place stuffed mushrooms on a baking sheet and bake in the preheated oven for 20-25 minutes, or until mushrooms are tender.

6. Garnish with fresh cilantro before serving.

Nutritional Value: Calories: 200 | Protein: 10g | Carbohydrates: 30g | Fats: 5g | Sodium: 150mg | Potassium: 300mg | Phosphorus: 150mg | Fiber: 8g

Tofu and Vegetable Stir-Fry with Brown Rice

Prep Time: 15 minutes | **Cook Time:** 15 minutes | **Total Time:** 30 minutes | **Per Serving:** 4 servings

Ingredients:

- 1 block (14 ounces) of firm tofu, drained and cubed

- 2 cups mixed vegetables (bell peppers, broccoli, snap peas, carrots), sliced

- 1 onion, sliced

- 2 cloves garlic, minced

- 2 tablespoons low-sodium soy sauce

- 1 tablespoon sesame oil

- 1 tablespoon rice vinegar

- 1 teaspoon ground ginger

- 4 cups cooked brown rice

Instructions:

1. In a large skillet, heat sesame oil over medium heat. Add cubed tofu and cook until golden brown on all sides. Remove from skillet and set aside.

2. In the same skillet, add sliced onion and minced garlic. Cook until softened.

3. Add mixed vegetables to the skillet and stir-fry until tender-crisp.

4. Return cooked tofu to the skillet.

5. In a small bowl, whisk together low-sodium soy sauce, rice vinegar, and ground ginger. Pour over tofu and vegetables in the skillet. Stir to combine and heat through.

6. Serve hot cooked brown rice.

Nutritional Value: Calories: 250 | Protein: 15g | Carbohydrates: 30g | Fats: 8g | Sodium: 200mg | Potassium: 300mg | Phosphorus: 200mg | Fiber: 5g

Roasted Vegetable and Hummus Wrap with Whole Grain Tortilla

Prep Time: 15 minutes | **Cook Time:** 20 minutes | **Total Time:** 35 minutes | **Per Serving:** 2 servings

Ingredients:

- 1 small zucchini, sliced
- 1 small yellow squash, sliced
- 1 red bell pepper, sliced
- 1 yellow bell pepper, sliced
- 1 small red onion, sliced
- 2 tablespoons olive oil
- Salt and pepper, to taste
- 1/2 cup low-sodium hummus
- 2 whole grain tortillas
- Fresh spinach leaves, for serving

Instructions:

1. Preheat oven to 400°F (200°C).
2. Place sliced zucchini, yellow squash, red bell pepper, yellow bell pepper, and red onion on a baking sheet.
3. Drizzle with olive oil and season with salt and pepper. Toss to coat.
4. Roast in the preheated oven for 15-20 minutes, or until vegetables are tender and caramelized.
5. Spread a layer of low-sodium hummus onto each whole-grain tortilla.
6. Top with roasted vegetables and fresh spinach leaves.
7. Roll up the tortillas and slice them in half.

Nutritional Value: Calories: 300 | Protein: 10g | Carbohydrates: 35g | Fats: 15g | Sodium: 200mg | Potassium: 400mg | Phosphorus: 150mg | Fiber: 8g

Lentil and Vegetable Shepherd's Pie with Mashed Cauliflower

Prep Time: 20 minutes | **Cook Time:** 40 minutes | **Total Time:** 1 hour | **Per Serving:** 4 servings

Ingredients:

- 2 cups cooked green or brown lentils
- 1 onion, diced
- 2 cloves garlic, minced
- 2 carrots, diced
- 1 cup green peas (fresh or frozen)
- 1 cup low-sodium vegetable broth
- 1 tablespoon tomato paste
- 1 teaspoon dried thyme
- Salt and pepper, to taste
- 1 head cauliflower, chopped
- 2 tablespoons unsweetened almond milk
- 1 tablespoon olive oil

Instructions:

1. Preheat oven to 375°F (190°C).

2. In a large skillet, sauté diced onion and minced garlic until softened.

3. Add diced carrots to the skillet and cook until slightly softened.

4. Stir in cooked lentils, green peas, low-sodium vegetable broth, tomato paste, dried thyme, salt, and pepper. Simmer for 10-15 minutes, until the mixture thickens.

5. Meanwhile, steam chopped cauliflower until very tender.

6. Transfer steamed cauliflower to a large bowl. Add unsweetened almond milk and olive oil. Mash until smooth.

7. Transfer the lentil and vegetable mixture to a baking dish.

8. Spread mashed cauliflower evenly over the lentil mixture.

9. Bake in the preheated oven for 20-25 minutes, or until the top is golden brown.

10. Serve hot.

Nutritional Value: Calories: 250 | Protein: 10g | Carbohydrates: 40g | Fats: 5g | Sodium: 200mg | Potassium: 400mg | Phosphorus: 200mg | Fiber: 12g

Chickpea and Vegetable Curry with Basmati Rice

Prep Time: 15 minutes | **Cook Time:** 30 minutes | **Total Time:** 45 minutes | **Per Serving:** 4 servings

Ingredients:

- 1 can (15 ounces) low-sodium chickpeas, drained and rinsed
- 2 cups mixed vegetables (bell peppers, carrots, peas), diced
- 1 onion, diced
- 2 cloves garlic, minced
- 1 tablespoon curry powder
- 1 teaspoon ground turmeric
- 1 teaspoon ground cumin
- 1 can (14 ounces) low-sodium diced tomatoes
- 1 can (14 ounces) light coconut milk
- Salt and pepper, to taste
- 2 cups cooked basmati rice

Instructions:

1. In a large skillet, sauté diced onion and minced garlic until softened.

2. Add diced mixed vegetables to the skillet and cook until tender.

3. Stir in curry powder, ground turmeric, and ground cumin. Cook for 1-2 minutes, until fragrant.

4. Add low-sodium diced tomatoes (with juices) and light coconut milk to the skillet. Bring to a simmer.

5. Add drained and rinsed chickpeas to the skillet. Simmer for 10-15 minutes to allow flavors to blend.

6. Season the curry with salt and pepper to taste.

7. Serve hot cooked basmati rice.

Nutritional Value: Calories: 300 | Protein: 10g | Carbohydrates: 50g | Fats: 8g | Sodium: 150mg | Potassium: 400mg | Phosphorus: 200mg | Fiber: 8g

Quinoa and Roasted Vegetable Bowl with Tahini Dressing

Prep Time: 15 minutes | **Cook Time:** 25 minutes | **Total Time:** 40 minutes | **Per Serving:** 4 servings

Ingredients:

- 1 cup quinoa, rinsed
- 2 cups mixed vegetables (bell peppers, zucchini, cherry tomatoes), diced
- 1 tablespoon olive oil
- Salt and pepper, to taste
- 1/4 cup tahini
- 2 tablespoons lemon juice
- 2 tablespoons water
- 1 clove garlic, minced
- Fresh parsley, for garnish

Instructions:

1. Preheat oven to 400°F (200°C).
2. In a large bowl, toss diced mixed vegetables with olive oil, salt, and pepper.
3. Spread vegetables in a single layer on a baking sheet.
4. Roast in the preheated oven for 20-25 minutes, or until tender and caramelized.
5. Meanwhile, cook quinoa according to package instructions.
6. In a small bowl, whisk together tahini, lemon juice, water, minced garlic, salt, and pepper to make the dressing.
7. To assemble the bowls, divide cooked quinoa among serving bowls. Top with roasted vegetables.
8. Drizzle with tahini dressing and garnish with fresh parsley.

Nutritional Value: Calories: 300 | Protein: 10g | Carbohydrates: 40g | Fats: 12g | Sodium: 100mg | Potassium: 300mg | Phosphorus: 150mg | Fiber: 8g

Tofu and Broccoli Stir-Fry with Brown Rice Noodles

Prep Time: 15 minutes | **Cook Time:** 15 minutes | **Total Time:** 30 minutes | **Per Serving:** 4 servings

Ingredients:

- 8 ounces brown rice noodles
- 1 block (14 ounces) of firm tofu, drained and cubed
- 2 cups broccoli florets
- 1 red bell pepper, sliced
- 1 yellow bell pepper, sliced
- 1/4 cup low-sodium soy sauce
- 2 tablespoons hoisin sauce
- 1 tablespoon sesame oil
- 2 cloves garlic, minced
- 1 teaspoon grated ginger
- Sesame seeds, for garnish

Instructions:

1. Cook brown rice noodles according to package instructions. Drain and set aside.

2. In a large skillet, heat sesame oil over medium heat. Add cubed tofu and cook until golden brown on all sides. Remove from skillet and set aside.

3. In the same skillet, add minced garlic and grated ginger. Cook until fragrant.

4. Add sliced bell peppers and broccoli florets to the skillet. Stir-fry until vegetables are tender-crisp.

5. Return cooked tofu to the skillet.

6. In a small bowl, whisk together low-sodium soy sauce and hoisin sauce. Pour over tofu and vegetables in the skillet. Stir to combine and heat through.

7. Serve hot cooked brown rice noodles, garnished with sesame seeds.

Nutritional Value: Calories: 300 | Protein: 15g | Carbohydrates: 40g | Fats: 8g | Sodium: 200mg | Potassium: 300mg | Phosphorus: 150mg | Fiber: 6g

Lentil and Sweet Potato Soup with Whole Grain Bread

Prep Time: 15 minutes | **Cook Time:** 30 minutes | **Total Time:** 45 minutes | **Per Serving:** 4 servings

Ingredients:

- 1 cup dry green or brown lentils, rinsed

- 2 sweet potatoes, peeled and diced

- 1 onion, diced

- 2 cloves garlic, minced

- 4 cups low-sodium vegetable broth

- 1 can (14 ounces) diced tomatoes

- 1 teaspoon ground cumin

- 1/2 teaspoon ground turmeric

- Salt and pepper, to taste

- 4 slices whole grain bread

Instructions:

1. In a large pot, combine rinsed lentils, diced sweet potatoes, diced onion, minced garlic, low-sodium vegetable broth, diced tomatoes (with juices), ground cumin, and ground turmeric.

2. Bring the soup to a boil, then reduce heat and simmer for 25-30 minutes, or until lentils and sweet potatoes are tender.

3. Season the soup with salt and pepper to taste.

4. Serve hot with whole-grain bread.

Nutritional Value: Calories: 250 | Protein: 10g | Carbohydrates: 40g | Fats: 5g | Sodium: 150mg | Potassium: 400mg | Phosphorus: 200mg | Fiber: 10g

Roasted Vegetable and Feta Stuffed Eggplant

Prep Time: 15 minutes | **Cook Time:** 40 minutes | **Total Time:** 55 minutes | **Per Serving:** 4 servings

Ingredients:

- 2 large eggplants
- 2 cups mixed vegetables (zucchini, bell peppers, cherry tomatoes), diced
- 1 onion, diced
- 2 cloves garlic, minced
- 2 tablespoons olive oil
- Salt and pepper, to taste
- 1/2 cup crumbled feta cheese
- Fresh parsley, for garnish

Instructions:

1. Preheat oven to 400°F (200°C).
2. Slice each eggplant in half lengthwise and scoop out the flesh, leaving about a 1/2-inch shell.
3. Chop the scooped-out eggplant flesh into small pieces.
4. In a large skillet, heat olive oil over medium heat. Add diced onion and minced garlic. Cook until softened.
5. Add diced mixed vegetables and chopped eggplant flesh to the skillet. Cook until vegetables are tender.
6. Season with salt and pepper to taste.
7. Fill each eggplant shell with the vegetable mixture.
8. Place stuffed eggplants on a baking sheet and bake in the preheated oven for 30-35 minutes, or until eggplants are tender.
9. Remove from oven and sprinkle crumbled feta cheese over the top of each stuffed eggplant.
10. Garnish with fresh parsley before serving.

Nutritional Value: Calories: 200 | Protein: 8g | Carbohydrates: 25g | Fats: 10g | Sodium: 150mg | Potassium: 400mg | Phosphorus: 150mg | Fiber: 10g

Side Dishes

Roasted Sweet Potatoes with Cinnamon

Prep Time: 10 minutes | **Cook Time:** 30 minutes | **Total Time:** 40 minutes | **Per Serving:** 4 servings

Ingredients:

- 2 large sweet potatoes, peeled and diced

- 1 tablespoon olive oil

- 1 teaspoon ground cinnamon

- Salt, to taste

Instructions:

1. Preheat oven to 400°F (200°C).

2. In a large bowl, toss diced sweet potatoes with olive oil, ground cinnamon, and salt until evenly coated.

3. Spread sweet potatoes in a single layer on a baking sheet.

4. Roast in the preheated oven for 25-30 minutes, or until tender and caramelized, stirring halfway through.

5. Serve hot.

Nutritional Value: Calories: 150 | Protein: 2g | Carbohydrates: 30g | Fats: 3g | Sodium: 50mg | Potassium: 400mg | Phosphorus: 80mg | Fiber: 5g

Steamed Broccoli with Garlic and Lemon

Prep Time: 10 minutes | **Cook Time:** 10 minutes | **Total Time:** 20 minutes | **Per Serving:** 4 servings

Ingredients:

- 4 cups broccoli florets
- 2 cloves garlic, minced
- 1 tablespoon olive oil
- 1 tablespoon lemon juice
- Salt and pepper, to taste

Instructions:

1. Place broccoli florets in a steamer basket.
2. Steam broccoli over boiling water for 5-7 minutes, or until tender-crisp.
3. In a small skillet, heat olive oil over medium heat. Add minced garlic and cook until fragrant.
4. Remove from heat and stir in lemon juice.
5. Drizzle garlic and lemon mixture over steamed broccoli.
6. Season with salt and pepper to taste.
7. Serve hot.

Nutritional Value: Calories: 50 | Protein: 2g | Carbohydrates: 5g | Fats: 3g | Sodium: 20mg | Potassium: 200mg | Phosphorus: 40mg | Fiber: 3g

Quinoa Tabbouleh with Parsley and Mint

Prep Time: 15 minutes | **Cook Time:** 15 minutes | **Total Time:** 30 minutes | **Per Serving:** 4 servings

Ingredients:

- 1 cup quinoa, rinsed

- 2 cups water

- 1 cup fresh parsley, chopped

- 1/2 cup fresh mint leaves, chopped

- 1/2 cup cherry tomatoes, halved

- 1/4 cup red onion, finely chopped

- 2 tablespoons olive oil

- 2 tablespoons lemon juice

- Salt and pepper, to taste

Instructions:

1. In a medium saucepan, bring water to a boil. Add quinoa, reduce heat to low, cover, and simmer for 15 minutes, or until quinoa is tender and water is absorbed. Remove from heat and let cool.

2. In a large bowl, combine cooked quinoa, chopped parsley, chopped mint leaves, halved cherry tomatoes, and finely chopped red onion.

3. In a small bowl, whisk together olive oil and lemon juice. Pour over the quinoa mixture and toss to combine.

4. Season with salt and pepper to taste.

5. Serve chilled or at room temperature.

Nutritional Value: Calories: 150 | Protein: 4g | Carbohydrates: 20g | Fats: 6g | Sodium: 20mg | Potassium: 150mg | Phosphorus: 80mg | Fiber: 3g

Roasted Brussels Sprouts with Balsamic Glaze

Prep Time: 10 minutes | **Cook Time:** 25 minutes | **Total Time:** 35 minutes | **Per Serving:** 4 servings

Ingredients:

- 1 pound Brussels sprouts, trimmed and halved
- 2 tablespoons olive oil
- Salt and pepper, to taste
- 2 tablespoons balsamic glaze

Instructions:

1. Preheat oven to 400°F (200°C).
2. In a large bowl, toss halved Brussels sprouts with olive oil, salt, and pepper until evenly coated.
3. Spread Brussels sprouts in a single layer on a baking sheet.
4. Roast in the preheated oven for 20-25 minutes, or until tender and caramelized, stirring halfway through.
5. Drizzle with balsamic glaze before serving.

Nutritional Value: Calories: 100 | Protein: 3g | Carbohydrates: 10g | Fats: 6g | Sodium: 20mg | Potassium: 300mg | Phosphorus: 80mg | Fiber: 4g

Cauliflower Rice Pilaf with Peas and Carrots

Prep Time: 10 minutes | **Cook Time:** 15 minutes | **Total Time:** 25 minutes | **Per Serving:** 4 servings

Ingredients:

- 1 head cauliflower, riced
- 1 cup frozen peas, thawed
- 1 cup diced carrots
- 1/2 onion, finely chopped
- 2 cloves garlic, minced
- 1 tablespoon olive oil
- 1/4 teaspoon ground cumin
- 1/4 teaspoon ground coriander
- Salt and pepper, to taste
- Fresh parsley, for garnish

Instructions:

1. In a food processor, pulse cauliflower florets until they resemble rice.
2. In a large skillet, heat olive oil over medium heat. Add finely chopped onion and minced garlic. Cook until softened.
3. Add diced carrots to the skillet and cook until slightly softened.
4. Stir in cauliflower rice, thawed peas, ground cumin, ground coriander, salt, and pepper.
5. Cook, stirring occasionally, for 5-7 minutes, or until cauliflower rice is tender.
6. Garnish with fresh parsley before serving.

Nutritional Value: Calories: 80 | Protein: 3g | Carbohydrates: 10g | Fats: 4g | Sodium: 30mg | Potassium: 300mg | Phosphorus: 60mg | Fiber: 4g

Grilled Asparagus with Lemon Zest

Prep Time: 5 minutes | **Cook Time:** 10 minutes | **Total Time:** 15 minutes | **Per Serving:** 4 servings

Ingredients:

- 1 pound asparagus, trimmed

- 1 tablespoon olive oil

- Zest of 1 lemon

- Salt and pepper, to taste

Instructions:

1. Preheat the grill to medium-high heat.

2. In a large bowl, toss trimmed asparagus with olive oil, salt, and pepper until evenly coated.

3. Place asparagus spears on the preheated grill and cook for 5-7 minutes, turning occasionally, until tender and lightly charred.

4. Remove grilled asparagus from the grill and transfer it to a serving platter.

5. Sprinkle with lemon zest before serving.

Nutritional Value: Calories: 30 | Protein: 2g | Carbohydrates: 5g | Fats: 2g | Sodium: 0mg | Potassium: 200mg | Phosphorus: 40mg | Fiber: 2g

Baked Zucchini Fries with Parmesan

Prep Time: 15 minutes | **Cook Time:** 20 minutes | **Total Time:** 35 minutes | **Per Serving:** 4 servings

Ingredients:

- 2 medium zucchinis, cut into fries
- 1/4 cup grated Parmesan cheese
- 1/4 cup whole grain breadcrumbs
- 1/2 teaspoon garlic powder
- 1/2 teaspoon dried oregano
- 1/4 teaspoon paprika
- Salt and pepper, to taste
- Cooking spray

Instructions:

1. Preheat oven to 425°F (220°C). Line a baking sheet with parchment paper and lightly coat with cooking spray.

2. In a shallow dish, combine grated Parmesan cheese, whole-grain breadcrumbs, garlic powder, dried oregano, paprika, salt, and pepper.

3. Dip zucchini fries into the breadcrumb mixture, pressing gently to adhere.

4. Place coated zucchini fries in a single layer on the prepared baking sheet.

5. Bake in the preheated oven for 18-20 minutes, or until golden brown and crisp.

6. Serve hot.

Nutritional Value: Calories: 60 | Protein: 4g | Carbohydrates: 8g | Fats: 2g | Sodium: 80mg | Potassium: 300mg | Phosphorus: 80mg | Fiber: 2g

Roasted Butternut Squash with Sage

Prep Time: 10 minutes | **Cook Time:** 30 minutes | **Total Time:** 40 minutes | **Per Serving:** 4 servings

Ingredients:

- 1 small butternut squash, peeled, seeded, and cubed

- 1 tablespoon olive oil

- 1 tablespoon chopped fresh sage

- Salt and pepper, to taste

Instructions:

1. Preheat oven to 400°F (200°C).

2. In a large bowl, toss cubed butternut squash with olive oil, chopped fresh sage, salt, and pepper until evenly coated.

3. Spread butternut squash in a single layer on a baking sheet.

4. Roast in the preheated oven for 25-30 minutes, or until tender and caramelized, stirring halfway through.

5. Serve hot.

Nutritional Value: Calories: 60 | Protein: 1g | Carbohydrates: 10g | Fats: 3g | Sodium: 0mg | Potassium: 300mg | Phosphorus: 40mg | Fiber: 3g

Sautéed Spinach with Garlic and Olive Oil

Prep Time: 5 minutes | **Cook Time:** 5 minutes | **Total Time:** 10 minutes | **Per Serving:** 4 servings

Ingredients:

- 1 tablespoon olive oil
- 2 cloves garlic, minced
- 8 cups fresh spinach leaves
- Salt and pepper, to taste

Instructions:

1. In a large skillet, heat olive oil over medium heat. Add minced garlic and cook until fragrant.
2. Add fresh spinach leaves to the skillet. Cook, stirring occasionally, until spinach is wilted.
3. Season with salt and pepper to taste.
4. Serve hot.

Nutritional Value: Calories: 30 | Protein: 2g | Carbohydrates: 2g | Fats: 2g | Sodium: 40mg | Potassium: 400mg | Phosphorus: 40mg | Fiber: 2g

Baked Sweet Potato Wedges with Rosemary

Prep Time: 10 minutes | **Cook Time:** 25 minutes | **Total Time:** 35 minutes | **Per Serving:** 4 servings

Ingredients:

- 2 medium sweet potatoes, scrubbed and cut into wedges

- 1 tablespoon olive oil

- 1 tablespoon chopped fresh rosemary

- Salt and pepper, to taste

Instructions:

1. Preheat oven to 425°F (220°C). Line a baking sheet with parchment paper.

2. In a large bowl, toss sweet potato wedges with olive oil, chopped fresh rosemary, salt, and pepper until evenly coated.

3. Spread sweet potato wedges in a single layer on the prepared baking sheet.

4. Bake in the preheated oven for 20-25 minutes, or until tender and lightly browned, flipping halfway through.

5. Serve hot.

Nutritional Value: Calories: 70 | Protein: 1g | Carbohydrates: 10g | Fats: 3g | Sodium: 20mg | Potassium: 200mg | Phosphorus: 40mg | Fiber: 2g

Snacks and Appetizers

Hummus with Carrot and Cucumber Sticks

Prep Time: 10 minutes | **Cook Time:** 0 minutes | **Total Time:** 10 minutes | **Per Serving:** 4 servings

Ingredients:

- 1 cup low-sodium canned chickpeas, drained and rinsed

- 2 tablespoons tahini

- 2 tablespoons lemon juice

- 1 clove garlic, minced

- 1/2 teaspoon ground cumin

- 1/4 teaspoon paprika

- Salt, to taste

- Carrot and cucumber sticks, for serving

Instructions:

1. In a food processor, combine chickpeas, tahini, lemon juice, minced garlic, ground cumin, paprika, and salt.

2. Process until smooth and creamy, adding water as needed to reach desired consistency.

3. Serve hummus with carrot and cucumber sticks.

Nutritional Value: Calories: 100 | Protein: 4g | Carbohydrates: 12g | Fats: 5g | Sodium: 70mg | Potassium: 150mg | Phosphorus: 80mg | Fiber: 4g

Roasted Chickpeas with Chili Lime Seasoning

Prep Time: 5 minutes | **Cook Time:** 25 minutes | **Total Time:** 30 minutes | **Per Serving:** 4 servings

Ingredients:

- 1 can (15 ounces) low-sodium canned chickpeas, drained and rinsed
- 1 tablespoon olive oil
- 1 teaspoon chili powder
- 1/2 teaspoon ground cumin
- 1/2 teaspoon garlic powder
- 1/2 teaspoon lime zest
- Salt, to taste

Instructions:

1. Preheat oven to 400°F (200°C). Line a baking sheet with parchment paper.
2. Pat dry the drained chickpeas with a paper towel.
3. In a bowl, toss chickpeas with olive oil, chili powder, ground cumin, garlic powder, lime zest, and salt until well coated.
4. Spread chickpeas in a single layer on the prepared baking sheet.
5. Roast in the preheated oven for 20-25 minutes, shaking the pan halfway through, until crispy.
6. Let cool before serving.

Nutritional Value: Calories: 120 | Protein: 5g | Carbohydrates: 15g | Fats: 4g | Sodium: 10mg | Potassium: 150mg | Phosphorus: 80mg | Fiber: 4g

Avocado Toast with Chia Seeds on Whole Grain Bread

Prep Time: 5 minutes | **Cook Time:** 0 minutes | **Total Time:** 5 minutes | **Per Serving:** 1 serving

Ingredients:

- 1 ripe avocado

- 2 slices low-sodium whole grain bread, toasted

- 1 tablespoon chia seeds

- Salt and pepper, to taste

Instructions:

1. Cut the avocado in half, remove the pit, and scoop the flesh into a bowl.

2. Mash the avocado with a fork until smooth.

3. Spread mashed avocado evenly onto the toasted whole-grain bread slices.

4. Sprinkle chia seeds over the avocado.

5. Season with salt and pepper, to taste.

6. Serve immediately.

Nutritional Value: Calories: 200 | Protein: 5g | Carbohydrates: 20g | Fats: 10g | Sodium: 100mg | Potassium: 300mg | Phosphorus: 100mg | Fiber: 8g

Baked Apple Chips with Cinnamon

Prep Time: 10 minutes | **Cook Time:** 2 hours | **Total Time:** 2 hours 10 minutes | **Per Serving:** 4 servings

Ingredients:

- 2 apples, cored and thinly sliced

- 1 teaspoon ground cinnamon

Instructions:

1. Preheat oven to 200°F (95°C). Line a baking sheet with parchment paper.

2. Arrange the apple slices in a single layer on the prepared baking sheet.

3. Sprinkle ground cinnamon over the apple slices.

4. Bake in the preheated oven for 2 hours, flipping the slices halfway through, until dried and crisp.

5. Let cool before serving.

Nutritional Value: Calories: 50 | Protein: 0g | Carbohydrates: 15g | Fats: 0g | Sodium: 0mg | Potassium: 100mg | Phosphorus: 10mg | Fiber: 3g

Edamame with Sea Salt

Prep Time: 5 minutes | **Cook Time:** 5 minutes | **Total Time:** 10 minutes | **Per Serving:** 4 servings

Ingredients:

- 2 cups frozen shelled edamame

- Sea salt, to taste

Instructions:

1. Bring a pot of water to a boil.

2. Add frozen shelled edamame to the boiling water and cook for 4-5 minutes, or until tender.

3. Drain the cooked edamame and transfer to a serving bowl.

4. Sprinkle with sea salt, to taste.

5. Serve hot or at room temperature.

Nutritional Value: Calories: 100 | Protein: 9g | Carbohydrates: 8g | Fats: 3g | Sodium: 0mg | Potassium: 200mg | Phosphorus: 100mg | Fiber: 4g

Celery Sticks with Peanut Butter

Prep Time: 5 minutes | **Cook Time:** 0 minutes | **Total Time:** 5 minutes | **Per Serving:** 1 serving

Ingredients:

- 2 celery stalks, cut into sticks

- 2 tablespoons low-sodium peanut butter

Instructions:

1. Spread peanut butter onto celery sticks.

2. Serve immediately.

Nutritional Value: Calories: 100 | Protein: 4g | Carbohydrates: 6g | Fats: 8g | Sodium: 70mg | Potassium: 200mg | Phosphorus: 80mg | Fiber: 3g

Roasted Red Pepper Dip with Whole Grain Crackers

Prep Time: 10 minutes | **Cook Time:** 25 minutes | **Total Time:** 35 minutes | **Per Serving:** 4 servings

Ingredients:

- 1 large red bell pepper

- 1/4 cup low-fat Greek yogurt

- 2 tablespoons lemon juice

- 1 clove garlic, minced

- 1 tablespoon chopped fresh parsley

- Salt and pepper, to taste

- Whole grain crackers, for serving

Instructions:

1. Preheat oven to 400°F (200°C). Line a baking sheet with parchment paper.

2. Place whole red bell pepper on the prepared baking sheet and roast in the preheated oven for 20-25 minutes, or until charred and tender.

3. Remove the roasted red bell pepper from the oven and let cool. Peel off the skin, remove the seeds, and chop the flesh.

4. In a food processor, combine chopped roasted red pepper, low-fat Greek yogurt, lemon juice, minced garlic, chopped fresh parsley, salt, and pepper. Blend until smooth.

5. Transfer the dip to a serving bowl and serve with whole-grain crackers.

Nutritional Value: Calories: 40 | Protein: 2g | Carbohydrates: 6g | Fats: 1g | Sodium: 40mg | Potassium: 120mg | Phosphorus: 40mg | Fiber: 1g

Cucumber Bites with Cream Cheese and Dill

Prep Time: 10 minutes | **Cook Time:** 0 minutes | **Total Time:** 10 minutes | **Per Serving:** 4 servings

Ingredients:

- 1 English cucumber, sliced

- 1/4 cup low-fat cream cheese

- 1 tablespoon chopped fresh dill

Instructions:

1. Spread a thin layer of low-fat cream cheese onto each cucumber slice.

2. Sprinkle chopped fresh dill over the cream cheese.

3. Serve immediately.

Nutritional Value: Calories: 30 | Protein: 1g | Carbohydrates: 2g | Fats: 2g | Sodium: 30mg | Potassium: 100mg | Phosphorus: 20mg | Fiber: 1g

Baked Zucchini Chips with Parmesan

Prep Time: 10 minutes | **Cook Time:** 25 minutes | **Total Time:** 35 minutes | **Per Serving:** 4 servings

Ingredients:

- 2 medium zucchinis, thinly sliced

- 1 tablespoon olive oil

- 2 tablespoons grated Parmesan cheese

- 1/2 teaspoon garlic powder

- Salt and pepper, to taste

Instructions:

1. Preheat oven to 425°F (220°C). Line a baking sheet with parchment paper.

2. In a large bowl, toss thinly sliced zucchini with olive oil, grated Parmesan cheese, garlic powder, salt, and pepper until evenly coated.

3. Arrange zucchini slices in a single layer on the prepared baking sheet.

4. Bake in the preheated oven for 20-25 minutes, or until golden brown and crispy.

5. Let cool before serving.

Nutritional Value: Calories: 50 | Protein: 2g | Carbohydrates: 3g | Fats: 3g | Sodium: 20mg | Potassium: 200mg | Phosphorus: 40mg | Fiber: 1g

Fruit Skewers with Honey Yogurt Dip

Prep Time: 10 minutes | **Cook Time:** 0 minutes | **Total Time:** 10 minutes | **Per Serving:** 4 servings

Ingredients:

- 1 cup low-fat Greek yogurt

- 1 tablespoon honey

- 1 teaspoon vanilla extract

- Assorted fruits (strawberries, pineapple, grapes, melon), cut into bite-sized pieces

- Wooden skewers

Instructions:

1. In a small bowl, whisk together low-fat Greek yogurt, honey, and vanilla extract until smooth.

2. Thread assorted fruit pieces onto wooden skewers.

3. Serve fruit skewers with honey yogurt dip.

Nutritional Value: Calories: 80 | Protein: 4g | Carbohydrates: 15g | Fats: 1g | Sodium: 20mg | Potassium: 150mg | Phosphorus: 80mg | Fiber: 2g

Desserts

Baked Apples with Cinnamon and Walnuts

Prep Time: 10 minutes | **Cook Time:** 30 minutes | **Total Time:** 40 minutes | **Per Serving:** 4 servings

Ingredients:

- 4 medium apples (such as Granny Smith or Honeycrisp), cored

- 2 tablespoons chopped walnuts

- 1 tablespoon honey

- 1/2 teaspoon ground cinnamon

- 1/4 teaspoon ground nutmeg

Instructions:

1. Preheat oven to 375°F (190°C).

2. Using a sharp knife, core the apples, leaving the bottom intact.

3. In a small bowl, mix chopped walnuts, honey, ground cinnamon, and ground nutmeg.

4. Stuff each apple with the walnut mixture.

5. Place stuffed apples in a baking dish and add a little water to the bottom of the dish.

6. Bake for 30 minutes, or until apples are tender.

7. Serve warm.

Nutritional Value: Calories: 120 | Protein: 1g | Carbohydrates: 25g | Fats: 3g | Sodium: 0mg | Potassium: 200mg | Phosphorus: 20mg | Fiber: 4g

Chia Pudding with Mango and Coconut Milk

Prep Time: 5 minutes | **Cook Time:** 0 minutes | **Total Time:** 5 minutes (+chilling time) | **Per Serving:** 2 servings

Ingredients:

- 1/4 cup chia seeds

- 1 cup unsweetened coconut milk

- 1 ripe mango, diced

- 2 tablespoons unsweetened shredded coconut (optional)

- 1 tablespoon honey or maple syrup (optional)

Instructions:

1. In a bowl, combine chia seeds and coconut milk. Stir well.

2. Cover and refrigerate for at least 2 hours or overnight, until the mixture thickens and resembles a pudding-like consistency.

3. To serve, layer chia pudding with diced mango in serving glasses or bowls.

4. Optional: Sprinkle with unsweetened shredded coconut and drizzle with honey or maple syrup.

5. Serve chilled.

Nutritional Value: Calories: 200 | Protein: 4g | Carbohydrates: 25g | Fats: 10g | Sodium: 10mg | Potassium: 200mg | Phosphorus: 80mg | Fiber: 10g

Roasted Pears with Honey and Ginger

Prep Time: 10 minutes | **Cook Time:** 25 minutes | **Total Time:** 35 minutes | **Per Serving:** 4 servings

Ingredients:

- 4 ripe pears, halved and cored

- 2 tablespoons honey

- 1 teaspoon ground ginger

- 1/4 teaspoon ground cinnamon

Instructions:

1. Preheat oven to 375°F (190°C).

2. Place pear halves on a baking sheet, and cut side up.

3. In a small bowl, mix honey, ground ginger, and ground cinnamon.

4. Drizzle the honey mixture over the pear halves.

5. Bake for 25 minutes, or until pears are tender and caramelized.

6. Serve warm.

Nutritional Value: Calories: 100 | Protein: 1g | Carbohydrates: 25g | Fats: 0g | Sodium: 0mg | Potassium: 200mg | Phosphorus: 20mg | Fiber: 4g

Frozen Banana Bites with Dark Chocolate

Prep Time: 10 minutes | **Cook Time:** 0 minutes | **Total Time:** 10 minutes (+freezing time) | **Per Serving:** 4 servings

Ingredients:

- 2 ripe bananas, peeled and sliced into rounds

- 1/4 cup dark chocolate chips

- 1 teaspoon coconut oil

- Chopped nuts or shredded coconut (optional)

Instructions:

1. Line a baking sheet with parchment paper.

2. Place banana slices on the prepared baking sheet.

3. In a microwave-safe bowl, combine dark chocolate chips and coconut oil. Microwave in 30-second intervals, stirring in between, until melted and smooth.

4. Dip each banana slice halfway into the melted chocolate, then place it back on the baking sheet.

5. Optional: Sprinkle with chopped nuts or shredded coconut.

6. Freeze for at least 1 hour, or until chocolate is set.

7. Serve frozen.

Nutritional Value: Calories: 100 | Protein: 1g | Carbohydrates: 20g | Fats: 3g | Sodium: 0mg | Potassium: 200mg | Phosphorus: 20mg | Fiber: 2g

Baked Cinnamon Apple Chips

Prep Time: 10 minutes | **Cook Time:** 2 hours | **Total Time:** 2 hours 10 minutes | **Per Serving:** 4 servings

Ingredients:

- 2 medium apples, cored and thinly sliced
- 1 teaspoon ground cinnamon

Instructions:

1. Preheat oven to 200°F (95°C). Line a baking sheet with parchment paper.
2. Arrange the apple slices in a single layer on the prepared baking sheet.
3. Sprinkle ground cinnamon over the apple slices.
4. Bake in the preheated oven for 2 hours, flipping the slices halfway through, until dried and crisp.
5. Let cool before serving.

Nutritional Value: Calories: 50 | Protein: 0g | Carbohydrates: 15g | Fats: 0g | Sodium: 0mg | Potassium: 100mg | Phosphorus: 10mg | Fiber: 3g

Coconut Chia Pudding with Berries

Prep Time: 5 minutes | **Cook Time:** 0 minutes | **Total Time:** 5 minutes (+chilling time) | **Per Serving:** 2 servings

Ingredients:

- 1/4 cup chia seeds

- 1 cup unsweetened coconut milk

- 1 tablespoon honey or maple syrup (optional)

- 1/2 teaspoon vanilla extract

- Mixed berries, for serving

Instructions:

1. In a bowl, combine chia seeds, coconut milk, honey or maple syrup (if using), and vanilla extract. Stir well.

2. Cover and refrigerate for at least 2 hours or overnight, until the mixture thickens and resembles a pudding-like consistency.

3. To serve, divide chia pudding into serving glasses or bowls.

4. Top with mixed berries.

5. Serve chilled.

Nutritional Value: Calories: 150 | Protein: 4g | Carbohydrates: 15g | Fats: 8g | Sodium: 10mg | Potassium: 100mg | Phosphorus: 80mg | Fiber: 9g

Grilled Peaches with Vanilla Greek Yogurt

Prep Time: 5 minutes | **Cook Time:** 5 minutes | **Total Time:** 10 minutes | **Per Serving:** 2 servings

Ingredients:

- 2 ripe peaches, halved and pitted
- 1/2 cup low-fat Greek yogurt
- 1 tablespoon honey
- 1/2 teaspoon vanilla extract

Instructions:

1. Preheat the grill to medium-high heat.
2. Place peach halves on the grill, cut side down, and grill for 3-4 minutes, or until grill marks appear.
3. In a small bowl, mix Greek yogurt, honey, and vanilla extract.
4. Serve grilled peaches with a dollop of vanilla Greek yogurt.

Nutritional Value: Calories: 100 | Protein: 5g | Carbohydrates: 20g | Fats: 1g | Sodium: 20mg | Potassium: 200mg | Phosphorus: 80mg | Fiber: 2g

Frozen Grapes with Lemon Zest

Prep Time: 5 minutes | **Cook Time:** 0 minutes | **Total Time:** 5 minutes (+freezing time) | **Per Serving:** 2 servings

Ingredients:

- 1 cup seedless grapes

- Zest of 1 lemon

Instructions:

1. Rinse grapes and pat dry with a paper towel.

2. Place grapes in a single layer on a baking sheet lined with parchment paper.

3. Sprinkle lemon zest over the grapes.

4. Freeze for at least 2 hours, or until grapes are firm.

5. Serve frozen.

Nutritional Value: Calories: 50 | Protein: 1g | Carbohydrates: 15g | Fats: 0g | Sodium: 0mg | Potassium: 100mg | Phosphorus: 10mg | Fiber: 1g

Baked Pear and Walnut Crisp

Prep Time: 10 minutes | **Cook Time:** 30 minutes | **Total Time:** 40 minutes | **Per Serving:** 2 servings

Ingredients:

- 2 ripe pears, peeled, cored, and sliced

- 1 tablespoon lemon juice

- 1/4 cup old-fashioned oats

- 2 tablespoons chopped walnuts

- 1 tablespoon honey or maple syrup

- 1/2 teaspoon ground cinnamon

- 1/4 teaspoon ground nutmeg

Instructions:

1. Preheat oven to 375°F (190°C).

2. In a bowl, toss pear slices with lemon juice.

3. In another bowl, combine oats, chopped walnuts, honey or maple syrup, ground cinnamon, and ground nutmeg.

4. Arrange pear slices in a baking dish and sprinkle the oat mixture over the top.

5. Bake for 25-30 minutes, or until the pears are tender and the topping is golden brown.

6. Serve warm.

Nutritional Value: Calories: 200 | Protein: 4g | Carbohydrates: 30g | Fats: 8g | Sodium: 0mg | Potassium: 200mg | Phosphorus: 80mg | Fiber: 6g

Coconut Milk Chia Pudding with Mango

Prep Time: 5 minutes | **Cook Time:** 0 minutes | **Total Time:** 5 minutes (+chilling time) | **Per Serving:** 2 servings

Ingredients:

- 1/4 cup chia seeds

- 1 cup unsweetened coconut milk

- 1 tablespoon honey or maple syrup (optional)

- 1/2 teaspoon vanilla extract

- 1 ripe mango, diced

Instructions:

1. In a bowl, combine chia seeds, coconut milk, honey or maple syrup (if using), and vanilla extract. Stir well.

2. Cover and refrigerate for at least 2 hours or overnight, until the mixture thickens and resembles a pudding-like consistency.

3. To serve, divide chia pudding into serving glasses or bowls.

4. Top with diced mango.

5. Serve chilled.

Nutritional Value: Calories: 200 | Protein: 4g | Carbohydrates: 25g | Fats: 10g | Sodium: 10mg | Potassium: 200mg | Phosphorus: 80mg | Fiber: 9g

Beverages

Infused Water with Cucumber and Mint

Prep Time: 5 minutes | **Cook Time:** 0 minutes | **Total Time:** 5 minutes | **Per Serving:** 1 serving

Ingredients:

- 1/2 cucumber, sliced

- 3-4 fresh mint leaves

- 2 cups water

- Ice cubes (optional)

Instructions:

1. In a pitcher, combine cucumber slices and fresh mint leaves.

2. Add water and stir to combine.

3. Refrigerate for at least 1 hour to allow the flavors to infuse.

4. Serve over ice cubes, if desired.

Nutritional Value: Calories: 0 | Protein: 0g | Carbohydrates: 0g | Fats: 0g | Sodium: 0mg | Potassium: 50mg | Phosphorus: 10mg | Fiber: 0g

Unsweetened Herbal Iced Tea

Prep Time: 5 minutes | **Cook Time:** 5 minutes | **Total Time:** 10 minutes (+chilling time) | **Per Serving:** 1 serving

Ingredients:

- 1 herbal tea bag (such as chamomile, peppermint, or hibiscus)

- 2 cups boiling water

- Ice cubes

- Fresh lemon slices (optional)

- Fresh mint leaves (optional)

Instructions:

1. Place the herbal tea bag in a heatproof pitcher.

2. Pour boiling water over the tea bag.

3. Let steep for 5 minutes, then remove the tea bag.

4. Refrigerate until chilled.

5. Serve over ice cubes with fresh lemon slices and mint leaves, if desired.

Nutritional Value: Calories: 0 | Protein: 0g | Carbohydrates: 0g | Fats: 0g | Sodium: 0mg | Potassium: 0mg | Phosphorus: 0mg | Fiber: 0g

Sparkling Water with Lemon and Lime

Prep Time: 5 minutes | **Cook Time:** 0 minutes | **Total Time:** 5 minutes | **Per Serving:** 1 serving

Ingredients:

- 1 cup sparkling water

- 1/2 lemon, sliced

- 1/2 lime, sliced

- Ice cubes (optional)

Instructions:

1. In a glass, combine sparkling water with lemon and lime slices.

2. Add ice cubes, if desired.

3. Stir gently to combine.

4. Serve immediately.

Nutritional Value: Calories: 0 | Protein: 0g | Carbohydrates: 0g | Fats: 0g | Sodium: 0mg | Potassium: 0mg | Phosphorus: 0mg | Fiber: 0g

Unsweetened Almond Milk with Cinnamon

Prep Time: 5 minutes | **Cook Time:** 0 minutes | **Total Time:** 5 minutes | **Per Serving:** 1 serving

Ingredients:

- 1 cup unsweetened almond milk

- 1/4 teaspoon ground cinnamon

Instructions:

1. In a glass, pour unsweetened almond milk.

2. Sprinkle ground cinnamon over the almond milk.

3. Stir gently to combine.

4. Serve immediately.

Nutritional Value: Calories: 30 | Protein: 1g | Carbohydrates: 1g | Fats: 3g | Sodium: 150mg | Potassium: 40mg | Phosphorus: 20mg | Fiber: 0g

Infused Water with Strawberry and Basil

Prep Time: 5 minutes | **Cook Time:** 0 minutes | **Total Time:** 5 minutes | **Per Serving:** 1 serving

Ingredients:

- 2-3 strawberries, sliced

- 2-3 fresh basil leaves

- 2 cups water

- Ice cubes (optional)

Instructions:

1. In a pitcher, combine sliced strawberries and fresh basil leaves.

2. Add water and stir to combine.

3. Refrigerate for at least 1 hour to allow the flavors to infuse.

4. Serve over ice cubes, if desired.

Nutritional Value: Calories: 0 | Protein: 0g | Carbohydrates: 0g | Fats: 0g | Sodium: 0mg | Potassium: 50mg | Phosphorus: 10mg | Fiber: 0g

Unsweetened Green Tea

Prep Time: 5 minutes | **Cook Time:** 5 minutes | **Total Time:** 10 minutes | **Per Serving:** 1 serving

Ingredients:

- 1 green tea bag

- 1 cup boiling water

Instructions:

1. Place the green tea bag in a cup.

2. Pour boiling water over the tea bag.

3. Let steep for 3-5 minutes, depending on desired strength.

4. Remove the tea bag and discard.

5. Serve hot.

Nutritional Value: Calories: 0 | Protein: 0g | Carbohydrates: 0g | Fats: 0g | Sodium: 0mg | Potassium: 0mg | Phosphorus: 0mg | Fiber: 0g

Sparkling Water with Grapefruit and Rosemary

Prep Time: 5 minutes | **Cook Time:** 0 minutes | **Total Time:** 5 minutes | **Per Serving:** 1 serving

Ingredients:

- 1/2 cup sparkling water
- 1/4 cup freshly squeezed grapefruit juice
- 1 sprig of fresh rosemary
- Ice cubes (optional)

Instructions:

1. In a glass, combine sparkling water with freshly squeezed grapefruit juice.
2. Add a sprig of fresh rosemary.
3. Add ice cubes, if desired.
4. Stir gently to combine.
5. Serve immediately.

Nutritional Value: Calories: 10 | Protein: 0g | Carbohydrates: 3g | Fats: 0g | Sodium: 0mg | Potassium: 70mg | Phosphorus: 10mg | Fiber: 0g

Unsweetened Coconut Water

Prep Time: 5 minutes | **Cook Time:** 0 minutes | **Total Time:** 5 minutes | **Per Serving:** 1 serving

Ingredients:

- 1 cup unsweetened coconut water

- Ice cubes (optional)

Instructions:

1. Pour unsweetened coconut water into a glass.

2. Add ice cubes, if desired.

3. Serve chilled.

Nutritional Value: Calories: 45 | Protein: 1g | Carbohydrates: 9g | Fats: 0g | Sodium: 40mg | Potassium: 470mg | Phosphorus: 20mg | Fiber: 0g

Infused Water with Blueberry and Thyme

Prep Time: 5 minutes | **Cook Time:** 0 minutes | **Total Time:** 5 minutes | **Per Serving:** 1 serving

Ingredients:

- 1/4 cup fresh blueberries
- 2-3 sprigs fresh thyme
- 2 cups water
- Ice cubes (optional)

Instructions:

1. In a pitcher, combine fresh blueberries and fresh thyme sprigs.
2. Add water and stir to combine.
3. Refrigerate for at least 1 hour to allow the flavors to infuse.
4. Serve over ice cubes, if desired.

Nutritional Value: Calories: 10 | Protein: 0g | Carbohydrates: 3g | Fats: 0g | Sodium: 0mg | Potassium: 30mg | Phosphorus: 10mg | Fiber: 1g

Unsweetened Chamomile Tea

Prep Time: 5 minutes | **Cook Time:** 5 minutes | **Total Time:** 10 minutes | **Per Serving:** 1 serving

Ingredients:

- 1 chamomile tea bag
- 1 cup boiling water

Instructions:

1. Place the chamomile tea bag in a cup.
2. Pour boiling water over the tea bag.
3. Let steep for 5 minutes.
4. Remove the tea bag and discard.
5. Serve hot.

Nutritional Value: Calories: 0 | Protein: 0g | Carbohydrates: 0g | Fats: 0g | Sodium: 0mg | Potassium: 0mg | Phosphorus: 0mg | Fiber: 0g

Measurement

Measurement	USA	UK	Europe
Volume			
1 teaspoon	1 tsp (4.93 mL)	1 tsp (5 mL)	1 tsp (5 mL)
1 tablespoon	1 tbsp (14.79 mL)	1 tbsp (15 mL)	1 tbsp (15 mL)
1 fluid ounce	1 fl oz (29.57 mL)	1 fl oz (28.41 mL)	1 fl oz (30 mL)
1 cup	1 cup (240 mL)	1 cup (284 mL)	1 cup (250 mL)
1 pint	1 pint (473 mL)	1 pint (568 mL)	1 pint (500 mL)
1 quart	1 quart (946 mL)	1 quart (1.136 L)	1 quart (1 L)
1 gallon	1 gallon (3.785 L)	1 gallon (4.546 L)	1 gallon (4 L)
Weight			
1 ounce	1 oz (28.35 g)	1 oz (28.35 g)	1 oz (28.35 g)
1 pound	1 lb (453.59 g)	1 lb (453.59 g)	1 lb (453.59 g)
Length			
1 inch	1 in (2.54 cm)	1 in (2.54 cm)	1 in (2.54 cm)
Temperature			
Freezing Point	32°F (0°C)	32°F (0°C)	32°F (0°C)
Boiling Point	212°F (100°C)	212°F (100°C)	212°F (100°C)

www.ingramcontent.com/pod-product-compliance
Lightning Source LLC
Chambersburg PA
CBHW081215260726
48653CB00010BA/3671